forgetting

MORE ADVANCE PRAISE FOR
FORGETTING: WHEN TO WORRY, WHAT TO DO

"As people age, memory loss is one of the most perplexing and mysterious areas of concern. Breitung explores and presents in a very readable manner the various forms of cognitive impairment. She addresses the symptoms and describes the various forms of memory problems. In her chapter on depression she points out the importance of diagnosis and treatment. She lists a wide range of services available to both the aging person as well as the caregiver. This is a book for both professionals and individuals caring for elderly family members and loved ones. . . . Deserves a place on the bookshelf of all who have aging parents, relatives, or friends."

**—Sr. Mary Caritas Geary, SP, former chair of the
Massachusetts Hospital Association**

". . . necessary reading for all of us as we age. A wonderful guide to what to look for, what is and what is not serious enough to seek treatment, and where to go for help. As our population ages, this [serves as] an outstanding how-to guide."

**—William A. Caplin, chartered life underwriter,
chartered financial consultant, and president,
board of directors, Greater Springfield, Massachusetts,
Senior Services**

forgetting

when to worry,
what to do

JOAN CARSON BREITUNG, RN, MSN

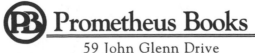

Prometheus Books

59 John Glenn Drive
Amherst, New York 14228–2119

Dedication

Jo Ben

Published 2008 by Prometheus Books

Inquiries should be addressed to
Prometheus Books
59 John Glenn Drive
Amherst, New York 14228–2119
VOICE: 716–691–0133, ext. 210
FAX: 716–691–0137
WWW.PROMETHEUSBOOKS.COM

12 11 10 09 08   5 4 3 2 1

Library of Congress Cataloging-in-Publication Data

Breitung, Joan Carson.
  Forgetting : when to worry, what to do / Joan C. Breitung.
      p. cm.
  Includes bibliographical references and index.
  ISBN 978–1–59102–617–4 (pbk. : alk. paper)
  1. Memory disorders in old age. 2. Older people—Health and hygiene. 3. Older people—Care. 4. Dementia. 5. Caregivers. I. Title. [DNLM: 1. Dementia—Popular Works. 2. Aged. 3. Caregivers—Popular Works. 4. Memory Disorders—Popular Works. 5. Physical Fitness—Popular Works. WM 75 B835f 2008]
  RC394.M46B74 2008
  616.8'3—dc22

                                                                    20080077759

Printed in the United States of America on acid-free paper

CONTENTS

Introduction

*L*ife expectancy in the United States is at an all-time high, and the average American can now expect to live approximately seventy-seven years. However, the blessings of greater longevity have generated their own peculiar set of problems and challenges. Although we are fortunate that medical science has improved our health and extended our lives, it is important to understand that age is the number-one risk factor for dementia. Old age is inextricably associated with this disorder, and forgetting is generally the first worrisome sign.

Forgetting: When to Worry, What to Do defines the kinds of memory problems that have straightforward explanations and remedies, as well as those that are more complex and ominous. This book stresses the importance of maintaining a reasonable level of physical fitness and emphasizes why a sedentary lifestyle can be a menace to both one's physical and cognitive health. It explains the compelling research that highlights the influence of dietary habits and the potential link between obesity and cognitive decline.

In order to emphasize the need for a prompt medical assessment when a memory problem interferes with someone's daily activities, chapter 1, "Reversible and Irreversible Dementia: Know Your

Enemy," defines the differences between reversible and irreversible dementias and lists the necessary steps people need to take to protect themselves physically and mentally. Practical strategies are suggested that can help boost cognitive reserve, the brain's ability to operate effectively even when its function is disrupted.

Technically, dementia is not an illness. It is a group of symptoms, chiefly memory loss, personality changes, behavioral problems, and the failure of other mental skills. Few disorders are more dreaded by older adults and their families than dementia because its alarming symptoms are precursors often of a future consisting of damaged minds, ruined relationships, total disability, and death.

Dementia is frequently confused with normal brain aging. Chapter 2, "Mild Cognitive Impairment: An Early Warning?" clarifies what the difference is and explains the two most familiar causes of cognitive impairment. Moreover, it describes another, lesser-known condition called mild cognitive impairment (MCI) that is an important feature in the spectrum of dementia. Many, but not all people with MCI progress to Alzheimer's disease (AD). Scientists still debate whether MCI is an early stage of AD, a distinct form of dementia, or a complex condition in which AD is one of several possible causes.

The most common dementia is Alzheimer's disease, and it is also the most feared consequence of aging. Chapter 3, "Alzheimer's Disease: Going, Going, Gone!" explains why and also warns of the future burden of the "mind thief," as some call this illness.

There are many situations in which what appears to be dementia is something else entirely. Most people are unaware that several common medical problems can be mistaken for dementia. Three illnesses that readily fall into this category are depression, delirium, and thyroid dysfunction. Fortunately, when these illnesses are diagnosed and treated correctly, the dementia is often reversed.

All healthcare professionals, however, are in agreement that Alzheimer's disease is by far the most prevalent dementing illness. It is a huge health issue because of its enormous impact on individuals, families, the healthcare system, and society as a whole. Since the aging population is growing, the incidence of AD is increasing. According to recent estimates, the number of older Americans with AD, now roughly 5 million, will soar dramatically as the population ages. Scientists are projecting that 11.3 million to 16 million individuals will be afflicted by 2050 unless new ways are found to prevent or treat the disease.

Former president Ronald Reagan's long public struggle with AD has led to a surge of interest in dementia, and in AD specifically. But all dementia is not AD. What is less well understood is that *everyone* is at risk for dementia since the major risk factor is old age. Furthermore, scientists have learned that there are other threats to cognition in addition to aging, and so they have stepped up the investigations of certain lifestyle habits and their links to these diseases. There is strong evidence, for example, that lifelong learning and mentally stimulating activities cannot only protect but also enhance our mental abilities.

Chapter 4, "Depression: More Than Just the Blues," addresses the illness of geriatric depression. An explanation of normal aging is compared with the symptoms of late-life depression and shows how the two are often confused. A stereotypical view of older adults is pervasive in our society. For example, elderly individuals who are withdrawn or apathetic may be showing signs of depression. Families, however, may think this conduct is an inevitable part of the aging process instead of a behavior that requires medical attention.

Families may despair when confronted with caring for someone with an irreversible disease. Yet just because an illness cannot be cured does not mean there is no treatment available. Caregiving responsibilities, stresses, and living arrangements are fully addressed in chapter 5, "Caregivers: Who Cares?" We list a wide range of resources for families faced with caring for a relative with an established dementia. These aids can help provide a better quality of life for both loved ones and caregivers.

As people with dementia gradually lose the ability to cope with their daily routines, they will need increasing supervision and hands-on assistance. Furthermore, as the disease progresses, they may develop alarming behaviors such as aggression, wandering, and paranoia. Consequently, it is not surprising that their caregivers become overwhelmed. In fact, studies have shown that caregivers in these situations experience higher levels of stress and depression than caregivers of terminally ill cancer patients. Learning about available resources provides caregivers with a measure of control and reassurance.

One of the oldest myths of aging is that normally, elderly persons lose their thinking abilities and the older a person becomes, the less alertness and competence can be expected. Chapter 6, "Dementia: Facts and Fiction," compares normal brain aging with several other neurological disorders and risks that can leave older adults susceptible to confusion and disorientation. For example, the elderly use more drugs because they have more illnesses than other individuals. *Polypharmacy*, the concurrent use of multiple drugs, is a common risk factor for confusion and lethargy since many drug side effects can cause symptoms similar to dementia. The consumption of multiple drugs because of numerous coexisting illnesses highlights the importance of drug reviews on a regular basis. This reinforces the underlying theme of the book, that although many elderly may be diagnosed with dementia, growing older is *not* the inevitable cause. Careful clinicians will take on the task of identifying behavioral changes that are true symptoms of dementia and conduct painstaking neuropsychological and physical assessments to arrive at an accurate diagnosis.

Chapter 7, "Falls: Accidents That Will Happen," explains why persons with dementia are at a much higher risk for falls and how to recognize potential environmental hazards inherent in various medical conditions common to older adults. A unique aspect of this chapter is the information about identifying and managing prominent risk factors that generally cause falls. Some examples are the importance of prompt treatment of visual problems, managing incontinence, and the close monitoring of the patient's medical regimen by both physician and caregiver.

Chapter 8, "Advice and Consent," promotes the belief that advance planning can help older adults make end-of-life decisions that are in their best interests. It explains the importance of having a will, describes end-of-life issues and choices, and emphasizes the necessity of advance directives.

Dementia is *never* part of normal aging. When forgetting and atypical behavior are interfering with everyday life, the situation should not be ignored. Denying this may be a useful coping mechanism for a short period of time, but prompt medical intervention is always in the patient's best interests. Unnecessary delay just makes a bad situation worse. As many health professionals warn, "Treatment delayed is treatment denied."

—J. C. B.

Chapter 1

Reversible and Irreversible Dementia

Know Your Enemy

*C*ognitive health is not static. When problems occur, they can range from mild cognitive impairment to severe dementia. We must understand that dementia is not a single disease but a collective term for numerous brain disorders that affect intellectual and social function, and to a great extent these interfere with the activities of daily living.

In the past, memory loss was viewed as one of the inevitable consequences of aging and it was often simply referred to as "senility." More recently, however, most clinicians have altered their view and now regard memory impairment of a certain degree as pathological (meaning caused by disease, from *pathology*, the study of disease) and indicative of a disease process that affects the brain.

A wide array of disorders that are increasingly found in older adults feature cognitive dysfunction as a common symptom. Identifying the reason for any mental deterioration is always essential for a person's health and well-being since studies show that there is a strong link between cognitive decline and an increase in illness and death (Gale 1996; McGlone 1990). The US Congressional Office of Technology Assessment estimates that as many as 6.8 million Americans suffer from some form of dementia, and at least 1.8 million of those 6.8 million are severely affected.

In studying dementia researchers have learned that some dementias overlap. A well-known example is when Alzheimer's disease and vascular dementia occur together. There are experts who believe this condition is very common. When an older adult becomes confused and forgetful, is unable to concentrate, or has difficulty with other thinking abilities, most people instinctively think of AD, the most common dementia. While there is no disputing that AD is the most prevalent dementing disorder—accounting for up to 70 percent of cases—there are many other disorders with symptoms of confusion and memory loss (AA 2005).

Even though it is common in very old individuals, dementia is not a normal part of the aging process and many people live into their nineties and even their hundreds without any cognitive impairment. It is worth noting that at the present time the majority of older adults do not experience dementia. Yet with older adults projected to represent an increasingly greater proportion of the US population, the cost of caring for people with cognitive impairments will become an increasingly weighty public health consideration.

Dementia is not a specific disease. Rather, it is a general term used to describe a group of symptoms that can be caused by a number of disorders that affect the brain. Such disorders include conditions that damage the brain's blood vessels or neurological structures. Individuals with dementia have characteristically impaired mental and behavioral functioning that hinders their normal activities and disrupts relationships. The most common feature among all these symptoms is memory loss. However, the loss of other intellectual abilities also occurs and is serious enough to interfere with daily life. Affected individuals also lose problem-solving abilities and emotional control. Other signs are changes in personality and behavior patterns such as agitation, delusions, and hallucinations. Although memory loss is a common indication, if it is the only symptom it should not be assumed that the affected individual has dementia.

Doctors diagnose dementia only if two or more brain functions—such as memory, language skills, perception, or cognitive skills including reasoning and judgment—are significantly impaired without loss of consciousness (NINDS 2006). This is why it is imperative to have an individual who shows early signs of increasing forgetfulness (or any other deterioration of intellectual function) medically evaluated before a dementia becomes full-blown. There are several types of cognitive decline that can be delayed or reversed with timely, appropriate treatment. Some conditions that can cause dementia, such as endocrine disorders, infections, vitamin deficiency, depression, and medication interactions, are treatable. Once the underlying causes of the dementia are treated, the situation often can be reversed.

Whether or not dementia is diagnosed as irreversible, an evaluation may uncover other treatable problems that might be compounding an individual's condition. Even irreversible forms of dementia can be treated with drugs to slow the advancing disease or modify behavioral problems.

CLASSIFYING DEMENTIAS

There are several satisfactory ways of classifying dementing disorders. One widely accepted method is to group illnesses together that have certain common characteristics, such as whether or not they will steadily worsen or what parts of the brain are affected. A widely accepted means of classifying dementias includes the following:

- Primary dementia: a dementia such as Alzheimer's disease, frontal lobe dementia, or Pick's disease that does not result from any other illness (Thackery 2006)
- Secondary dementia: a dementia that may be secondary or related to ingested substances, for example, alcohol, drugs, or toxins; infections; structural brain disorders (including normal pressure hydrocephalus), or to other potentially reversible disorders (Merck 2006)

There are several reasons dementing disorders can be very diffi-cult to recognize. Characteristically, the symptoms are insidious, starting slowly and not readily reflecting the harm being caused. To further complicate their identification, there may be episodes of normal behavior interspersed with obvious symptoms of cognitive decline as the disease progresses. Another barrier to prompt diagnosis is the ability of many individuals with dementia to temporarily hide or mask their symptoms during a physician's evaluation. Nevertheless, a complete medical assessment is absolutely essential because in time, the affected individuals can become so impaired that their very lives are threatened.

Advanced age has always been associated with medical issues as well as with normal, age-related cognitive decline. But memory loss problems seem to be the most common general complaint of seniors (Derouesne 1989; Nielson 2005). Practicing physicians know that it can be a challenge to distinguish between the normal changes in an older patient's cognitive functioning and those declines in thinking abilities that are related to disease, particularly if the patient's focus is on physical complaints.

Ordinarily, like anyone else, older adults have varying levels of intellectual skills. However, there are certain shared features that are associated with greater than average age-related changes in their thinking. These include low levels of education, genetic predisposition, hypertension, inactivity, and poor physical health (Christensen 2001).

PROMINENT IRREVERSIBLE DEMENTIAS

Alzheimer's disease is irreversible and it accounts for 50 to 60 percent of all dementing illnesses. Vascular dementias (for example, major cerebrovascular events known as strokes or "brain attacks," or microvascular pathology often called "ministrokes") are common in 15 to 20 percent of patients, and often occur with AD (Adelman and Daly 2005). AD is fully addressed in chapter 3.

Vascular Dementia

Vascular dementia (VaD), which is sometimes referred to as multi-infarct dementia, is the second most common form, ranking after AD and accounting for up to 20 percent of all dementias (Kalaria 2002). It is likely to have an increasingly negative impact on an expanding aging population.

VaD is caused by reduced blood flow to parts of the brain due to cerebrovascular or cardiovascular problems, usually strokes. VaD also may result from genetic diseases, endocarditis (inflammation of the lining of the heart and its valves), or amyloid angiopathy (a process in which a waxy substance called amyloid, composed mostly of protein, builds up in the brain's blood vessels, at times causing hemorrhagic strokes). It is important to note, however, that VaD can develop in the absence of strokes. It may also occur when the blood supply carrying oxygen and nutrients to the brain is interrupted by a blocked or diseased vascular system.

In many cases, VaD may coexist with AD. Up to one-fifth of people with AD may also be suffering from VaD. This is known as "mixed dementia." The incidence of vascular dementia increases with advancing age and is similar in men and women. Early detection and accurate diagnosis are important, as VaD is at least partially preventable. Some of the causes of vascular dementia are untreated hypertension, smoking, elevated cholesterol, diabetes, and heart disease. The immediate cause—what triggers the onset—is a stroke, a sudden interruption in the blood flow to the brain. There are two kinds of stroke. *Ischemic stroke*, the most common type, results from clogged arteries. *Hemorrhagic stroke*, bleeding in the brain, is the second most common type of stroke. It occurs when small blood vessels in the brain weaken and rupture. Although there is no treatment that can reverse the brain damage caused by a stroke, the prevention of future strokes is of major importance.

The symptoms of vascular dementia are often of sudden onset, typically appearing within three months after a stroke. Patients may have had a history of high blood pressure, vascular disease, or previous strokes or heart attacks. Worsening of VaD depends on whether or not the individual has additional strokes. In some cases symptoms may diminish. When the disease progresses it does so in a fluctuating, stepwise manner, with an abrupt deterioration of abilities, rather than the slow and steady decline usually seen in AD. However, there are also cases of VaD that seem to cause a gradual, more widespread cognitive impairment that looks very much like AD. Unlike people with AD, individuals with VaD often maintain their personality and customary levels of emotional responsiveness until the later stages of the disease. Patients with VaD do tend to wander at night and usually have other problems that are widespread among stroke victims such as depression, gait impairment, and incontinence. These symptoms also point to a vascular disorder rather than a degenerative illness (Roman et al. 1993).

A subtype of VaD is multi-infarct dementia (MID), which is caused by several small strokes in the brain. MID consists of multiple damaged areas, called infarcts, and extensive lesions due to a series of "ministrokes" that often go unnoticed. This results in damaging the area of the brain associated with learning, memory, and language. These ministrokes are sometimes referred to as transient ischemic attacks (TIAs), which result in only temporary and partial blockages of blood supply, causing brief impairments in consciousness or sight. TIA symptoms, which usually occur suddenly, are similar to those of stroke but do not last as long. Most of the symptoms disappear within an hour, although in some situations they may persist for up to twenty-four hours.

TIAs are often warning signs that a person is at risk for a more serious and debilitating stroke. About one-third of those who have a TIA will have an acute stroke, or a brain attack, sometime in the future. Many strokes can be prevented by heeding the warning signs of TIAs and treating the underlying risk factors.

Over time the damage caused to brain tissue will interfere with basic cognitive functions and disrupt everyday functioning. This happens because the infarcts affect isolated areas of the brain. Consequently, the symptoms are often limited to one side of the body and affect a single function such as language. A patient affected this way may understand language yet be unable to speak. Such a symptom is termed *local* or *focal*. Patients who neither understand language or are able to speak are said to be exhibiting *global symptoms*.

The symptoms of a TIA are often slight and in many cases, barely noticeable. They may include mild weakness in an arm or a leg, slurred speech, dizziness, and visual disturbance. All individuals who sustain a TIA need immediate medical attention.

Although not all strokes generate mental deficits, there are some situations in which a single stroke will damage the brain enough to do so. This can occur when one large vascular lesion causes severe brain damage, or when there is a single infarction in a strategic area of the brain. It is more common when the stroke occurs in the left hemisphere of the brain or when it involves the hippocampus—a key brain structure essential for memory.

A less frequently seen form of vascular dementia is Binswanger's disease. This illness is sometimes referred to as a subcortical dementia. It is a rare dementia characterized by cerebrovascular lesions in the deep white matter of the brain that causes losses of memory and cognition, as well as mood changes. Strokes are often a feature (Roman 1987). This uncommon disorder is a slowly progressive, irreversible condition for which there is no cure.

Diabetes, cardiac disease, previous cerebrovascular accident, malnutrition, and most notably hypertension have been associated with dementia of the Binswanger's type (McQuinn and O'Leary 1987; Olsen and Clasen 1998). Other hallmarks of the disease include urinary incontinence, difficulty walking, clumsiness, slowness of conduct, lack of facial expression, and speech difficulty. These symptoms, which tend to begin after the age of sixty, are not all present in every patient. Furthermore, they may sometimes appear only as a passing phase. The treatment for this type of dementia is symptomatic, meaning it involves treating the body's responses to the dementia, in this case primarily through the use of medications for controlling arrhythmias (abnormal heart rhythms), blood pressure, and depression. There are implications that control of hypertension may slow progression of the disease and aspirin therapy may prevent future cerebral infarcts. Consequently, the treatment consists of controlling hypertension and the appropriate use of aspirin prophylaxis, meaning taking a regiment of aspirin as a preventative measure (Olsen and Clasen 1998).

Another uncommon vascular dementia is linked to abnormalities of a specific gene located on chromosome 19. CADASIL, which stands for cerebral autosomal dominant arteriopathy, is a common form of hereditary disease of the arteries causing brain infarcts and dementia (Kalimo et al. 2002). This condition can cause multi-infarct dementia as well as stroke, mood disorders, and migraine with aura. An aura is a visual disturbance such as flashing or zigzagging lights or another type of visual hallucination.

Its varying symptoms make CADASIL difficult to diagnose and it is now believed to be more common than originally thought (Kalaria et al. 2002). Due to the high incidence of migraines in the population, CADASIL is often overlooked as a potential cause and may therefore not be diagnosed until the first stroke, a symptom rather commonly associated with CADASIL (Lesnik Oberstein et al. 2003).

There are several other causes of VaD, chiefly vasculitis (inflammation of a lymph or blood vessel), profound hypotension, or lesions that are triggered by a brain hemorrhage. The autoimmune disease lupus erythematosus—which causes skin damage, sometimes fatally—and the inflammatory disease temporal arteritis can damage blood vessels in a manner that brings about vascular dementia.

Vasculitis is an inflammation of the blood vessel system, which includes the veins, arteries, and capillaries. Any blood vessel is vulnerable. The symptoms of vasculitis depend on which blood vessels are involved and what organs in the body are affected.

Vasculitis may occur alone or with other disorders such as temporal arteritis. Temporal arteritis (also called cranial or giant cell arteritis) is an inflammation of the temporal artery that runs over the temple, beside the eye. The prognosis for individuals with vasculitis varies depending on the severity of the disorder (NINDS 2006).

> Dementias that can be reversed are far fewer than previously thought. While concurrent illnesses should always be treated for their own sake and in the hope that cognitive decline may at least be delayed, these present findings have significant clinical and economic implications (Clarfield 2003).

Lewy Body Dementia

Dementia with Lewy bodies is a neurodegenerative disorder associated with abnormal structures of protein (Lewy bodies) that form inside nerve cells in areas of the brain that govern thinking and movement. It often starts with wide variations in attention and alertness. While there have been rare familial cases reported, Lewy body dementia (LBD) usually occurs randomly in people with no known family history of the disease.

LBD is increasingly acknowledged as one of the more common forms of degenerative dementia and is difficult to diagnose. Some experts believe LBD is related to Alzheimer's disease or the form of Parkinson's disease associated with dementia. However, the emerging consensus is that LBD is a distinct pathologic entity somewhere between the two (Neef and Walling 2006). There are a variety of medical, neurological, and neuropsychological tests used to identify LBD and its possible overlap with other illnesses.

Symptoms can range from traditional parkinsonian effects, such as the loss of spontaneous movement, rigidity, tremor, and shuffling gait, to the shared warning signs of Alzheimer's disease: acute confusion, memory loss, and fluctuating cognition. There is considerable overlapping of symptoms. Visual hallucinations may be one of the first indications, and patients often develop other psychiatric disturbances such as delusions and depression. Typically, the onset of the disorder occurs in older adults, although younger people can be affected as well.

Treatment of LBD is symptomatic and it often involves using medication to control the parkinsonian and psychiatric symptoms. However, patients and their caregivers need to be aware the antiparkinsonian medication that can help to reduce tremors and loss of muscle movement has, in some cases, worsened some other problems such as delusions and hallucinations.

Doctors tend to avoid prescribing antipsychotics for hallucinatory symptoms of LBD because of the risk that sensitivity to these drugs could worsen the motor symptoms. Such drugs have even been associated with increased mortality. Cholinesterase inhibitor drugs are the mainstay of treatment for cognitive impairment. This class of drugs has also shown therapeutic benefit in reducing hallucinations and other neuropsychiatric symptoms of the disease. They are recommended as first-line therapy for the treatment of psychosis in LBD (Fernandez et al. 2003).

Frontotemporal Dementia

Frontotemporal dementia (FTD), sometimes called frontal lobe dementia, describes a group of diseases characterized by the degeneration of nerve cells, particularly those in the frontal and temporal lobes of the brain. Unlike Alzheimer's disease, frontotemporal dementia usually does not include formation of amyloid plaques. For many people with FTD there is an abnormal form of tau protein (a form of protein mostly present in the neurons in the brain), which amasses into neurofibrillary tangles commonly found in degenerating nerve cells. These structures disrupt normal cell activity and may cause cell death.

Researchers believe that FTD accounts for between 2 and 10 percent of all cases of dementia (Barker et al. 2002; NINDS 2004). The symptoms usually appear between the ages of forty and sixty-five, and the fact that in many instances there was or had been a family history of dementia suggests there is a strong genetic factor to the disease. The duration of FTD varies with some patients; some decline rapidly over two to three years while others show only minimal changes for many years. On average, people with FTD live for five to ten years after diagnosis.

Since structures found in the frontal and temporal lobes of the brain govern personality, judgment, planning, and organization, patients with frontotemporal dementia are often limited in their ability to maintain socially acceptable behavior and normal interactions with people. They display personality changes and general disorientation before exhibiting memory loss. Consequently, those afflicted with a frontotemporal dementia may, at times, act rudely and in an uninhibited and socially inappropriate manner. Patients are generally insensitive, indifferent to hygiene, and may be sexually aggressive. Other common symptoms include speech and language deficits, compulsive or repetitive behavior, increased appetite, and motor problems such as stiffness and difficulty maintaining balance. If memory loss occurs it generally happens later in the disease.

One type of FTD is Pick's disease in which the frontal and temporal lobes are most affected. Microscopically, certain nerve cells are found to have become swollen or balloon shaped. These distended neurons are hallmarks of the disease. The brains of those afflicted with Pick's disease also have abnormal structures within the neurons made up of tau protein that are called Pick bodies.

The symptoms of Pick's disease may overlap with Alzheimer's disease, however, there are a few distinct differences. First, the onset is earlier, taking place between forty and sixty years of age. Contrasted with AD, in which memory loss is the initial sign, the first symptom of the patient with Pick's disease typically is a personality change. Symptoms may range from restlessness to extreme apathy, overeating, hypersexuality, and general indifference to former interests. Generally, function declines because the patient simply does very little, or displays confusion and poor judgment. The disease is progressive and treatment is focused on managing symptoms and maximizing the individual's quality of life.

Although the cause of Pick's disease is unknown, it does run in some families and is thought to be genetic. At this time there is no way to slow the progressive degeneration of the illness. Nevertheless, medication is often helpful in treating depression, reducing aggression, and moderating other behavioral problems.

Another type of FTD that may begin in people as early as their forties is primary progressive aphasia (PPA), a dementia evidenced by problems with language. *Aphasia* is a general term applied to deficits in language function such as speaking, understanding speech, and naming common household objects. Individuals with PPA develop impairments in one or more of these functions.

This dementia is diagnosed when there has been progressive decline in language function for two or more years. Although activities of daily living are managed rather well during the first years of the disease, patients with primary progressive aphasia may lose the ability to care for themselves six to seven years after onset (Mendez et al. 1993).

The disease is subtle initially, with symptoms starting gradually then progressing very slowly over a period of years. As the course of disease evolves, memory and attention may also be damaged and patients could show alterations in personality and behavior. Eventually, most patients fully develop symptoms of dementia.

HIV/AIDS Dementia

This type of dementia results from an infection with the human immunodeficiency virus that destroys the brain's white matter. Typically, it is marked by apathy, faulty memory, inability to concentrate, and social withdrawal. Patients often develop movement difficulties as well. Although there is no specific treatment, AIDS drugs can delay the onset of the disease and may well help to diminish symptoms.

Huntington's Disease

Huntington's disease (HD) is a genetic disorder that causes widespread damage in many regions of the brain and spinal cord. The symptoms generally begin when patients are in their thirties or forties, and the average life expectancy after diagnosis is about fifteen years. Death is usually due to pneumonia, cardiopulmonary disease, trauma, or suicide (Sharon et al. 2005).

The cognitive symptoms of HD commonly begin with mild personality changes such as irritability, anxiety, and depression and progress to severe dementia. Many patients also develop psychoses. Chorea, the bizarre involuntary movements of the arms, legs, and facial muscles, is the primary physical symptom of HD followed by gait disturbances and general muscle weakness. Children of those who have the disease have a 50 percent chance of inheriting it.

Dementia Pugilistica

Dementia pugilistica (DP) is also known as chronic traumatic encephalopathy, or more commonly as boxer's syndrome. It is a memory disorder caused by head trauma. Such injuries are sustained when an individual is subjected to repeated blows to the head. Identical abnormal tau proteins, which form fibrous tangles in the brains of those stricken with AD, are found in patients with dementia pugilistica. Both diseases are marked by similar physical and memory disorders. However, this does not mean the diseases are the same. Although they share similar pathology, the fibrous lesions in AD and DP are generally found in different parts of the brain (Schmidt et al. 2001). The most common symptoms of the condition are dementia and parkinsonism (meaning Parkinson's disease or a neurological disorder resembling it), both of which can appear many years after the trauma ends.

It is also possible for a single traumatic brain injury to lead to a disorder called post-traumatic dementia. This disorder resembles dementia pugilistica, but it also includes long-term memory problems. Other symptoms vary depending on which part of the brain is injured.

Creutzfeldt-Jakob Disease

Creutzfeldt-Jacob disease (CJD) is a rare, rapidly degenerative fatal brain disorder that affects about one in every million people per year worldwide. The symptoms usually begin after age sixty and most patients die within one year. Many researchers believe that CJD is caused by a prion, a rogue form of protein. Most cases occur sporadically, that is, in people who have no known risk factors for the disease. However, about 5 to 10 percent of occurrences in the United States are hereditary and are caused by a mutation in the gene for the prion protein. In rare situations, CJD can also be acquired through exposure to diseased brain or nervous system tissue, usually through certain medical procedures. There is no evidence to suggest that this illness is airborne or that it is contagious through casual contact with a CJD patient.

CJD belongs to a family of human and animal diseases known as the transmissible spongiform encephalopathies (TSEs). Spongiform refers to the characteristic appearance of infected brains, which become filled with holes until they resemble sponges when viewed microscopically (NINDS 2006).

In recent years a variant of CJD has been found in Great Britain and several other European countries. The variant occurs in much younger patients, and the research strongly suggests that infections resulted from consumption of beef from cattle with bovine spongiform encephalopathy (BSE), also dubbed mad cow disease.

REVERSIBLE DEMENTIAS

Some dementias are partially or completely reversible when the underlying illness causing the dementia is treated. An example is normal pressure hydrocephalus (NPH), an uncommon, yet largely treatable dementia. The disease is caused by an accumulation of fluid in the brain and the cause is often unclear. Selected patients with NPH may be helped by surgery that drains the excess fluid.

Unfortunately, however, fewer than 10 percent of dementias are caused by treatable conditions (Adelman and Daly 2005). Although the percentage of reversible dementia is small when compared to the total number of dementias, it is still an urgent matter to identify and treat any causes of a potentially reversible dementia (Wivel 1988).

New interventions are also often helpful in forestalling further decline in functioning among people with a nonreversible dementia. Thus, a timely evaluation by a physician is key to optimal care of individuals with either a reversible or irreversible dementia.

Among the more frequent causes of reversible dementia are drug toxicity, depression, and alcohol abuse. Of all the problems older people face when taking medication, drug interactions that cause adverse events are probably the most dangerous. When two or more drugs are mixed in the body, they have the potential to interact with each other and produce uncomfortable or even dangerous side effects. As the average older person is taking more than four prescription medications concurrently plus two over-the-counter (OTC) medications, the risks for problems increase (FDA 2003). The adverse effects of polypharmacy, the taking of multiple drugs, is a common cause of cognitive decline.

Other causes of reversible cognitive decline are vitamin deficiencies, infections, thyroid dysfunction, and neurodegenerative and metabolic disorders (Espino et al. 1998). With appropriate treatment, the outcome is frequently successful. The presence of the following disorders need to be investigated before a confirmed diagnosis of irreversible dementia is made.

To help distinguish reversible dementias from potentially irreversible dementia, the use of the following mnemonic, DEMENTIA, which highlights the causes of reversible dementia, may prove helpful (Gambert 1997).

> **D** rugs and alcohol
> **E** motional disorders
> **M** etabolic and endocrine disorders
> **E** yes and ears
> **N** utritional deficiencies/normal pressure hydrocephalus
> **T** umors and trauma
> **I** nfections
> **A** rteriosclerosis

Drugs and Older Adults

People sixty-five and older represent 13 percent of the population, but they consume about 33 percent of all prescription medications (Williams 2002). Furthermore, new research reveals that one-third of seniors are taking medications prescribed by two or more physicians and that seven out of ten seniors report taking medications that were first prescribed for them more than six months ago (ASHP 2001).

Older patients are more likely to be prescribed multiple prescriptions for a long period of time. This often leads to unintentional misuse. Medication use in older adults requires special attention because of the increasing amount of drugs used by this group and the age-related changes in the body that affects how the drug is metabolized, or processed by the body.

Related factors recognized for placing the elderly at increased risk for adverse drug reactions include physiological changes caused by aging, chronic disease conditions, drug to drug interactions, and noncompliance with drug therapy. Since there is no universally accepted definition of polypharmacy, many clinicians simply use the term "prescription of more drugs than is clinically justified" to describe the practice (Reid 2005). Adverse reactions are not limited to the use of prescription drugs but also include OTC and herbal medicines, as well as vitamins and other supplements.

Cognitive disorders are one of the major risks of polypharmacy.

Others include an increase in the number of potentially inappropriate prescriptions, falls, hip fractures, depression, and incontinence (Rancourt et al. 2004). For more information on polypharmacy and falls, please see chapter 7.

Twenty-one studies of multiple medication use by older adults who live independently found that up to 27 percent of these elders were prescribed medications on the Beers List of Drugs. The Beers List describes drugs that may be inappropriate for elders because they were found to be ineffective or because the possibility for adverse effects is greater than the likelihood for benefit (Beers et al. 1991; Beers 1997; Wilkinson and Moskowitz 2001). Forty-eight medications or classes of drugs to avoid prescribing to adults sixty-five or older have recently been identified by a national expert panel charged with updating widely used criteria for potentially harmful medications in older adults (Fick, Cooper, and Wade 2003).

In most studies of elders' drug use, women are found to be using more medicines than men. Exactly why this occurs is unclear. However, the evidence suggests that women over eighty-five do indeed have more disabling ailments than men, mainly attributable to the higher prevalence of fractures and other bone- and joint-related disorders they sustain. This may also explain why women use more analgesics and sedatives/hypnotics than men (Correa-de-Araujo, Miller, and Banthin 2005).

The simultaneous use of multiple medications is a widely acknowledged cause of cognitive decline in elderly persons. Unfortunately, most patients and their families are unaware of just how much this practice increases the risk of adverse drug reactions or just how difficult it is going to be for the patient to comply satisfactorily with a medication regimen. It is enough of a challenge to avoid the effects of two or three interacting drugs, but when eight or ten of these potentially interacting compounds are used, it becomes virtually impossible to calculate the consequences.

Older adults are often taking prescriptions such as antidepressants, antiarrhythmics, antihypertensives, analgesics, and derivatives of digitalis, a cardiac drug that slows and strengthens the heart rate. It increases the flow of blood throughout the body. Combinations of any two of them can produce a reaction that is usually more forceful than for a younger individual. Examples of drug effects that are intensified is this manner are postural hypotension (a rapid drop in blood pressure when changing body position) with medications that lower blood pressure, dehydration and electrolyte imbalance when taking diuretics, bleeding complications with oral anticoagulants (drugs that aid in blood clotting), and gastrointestinal irritation with nonsteroidal anti-inflammatory drugs.

In general, elders are more sensitive to the effects of drugs than younger people because the elderly metabolize drugs much more slowly. Thus, the action of a drug may be magnified or longer lived in its effects, necessitating the adjustment of drug choice and dosage (Turnheim 2003).

AGING AS IT AFFECTS DRUG METABOLISM

Although the effects of aging on human drug metabolism has been studied by many researchers, few generalizations about how aging impacts human drug metabolism have emerged. However, the following are principles that have been established through research.

- Aging initiates a decline in kidney function. This affects the elimination of many drugs, increasing their half life, or the time it takes for the body to process half of a dosage.
- Aging bodies have less water and proportionately more fat, which affects the required dosage of drugs that are either water or fat soluble. This can lower the normal distribution of a drug within the body. Thus the drug will remain in the system for a longer period of time. For example, digoxin, a water-soluble drug used to treat heart conditions, would require that a lower dose be prescribed. A fat-soluble drug such as diazepam (better known as

Valium, used to treat anxiety) will encounter an
volume of distribution and thus result in a longer half lin
drug. This consequence will prolong the action of the drug.

- The aging process significantly changes the central nervous system. For example, there is a decline in our neurotransmitters, which relay information between our neurons and other cells. One form of neurotransmitter is acetylcholine. Neurons that contain acetylcholine are found in areas of the brain involved in memory, learning, and thinking. The circuits that connect these regions are powered by acetylcholine. If there is not enough of this compound available to the neurons, mental functions will become impaired, leading to dementia.
- Older adults are more vulnerable to prolonged and increased sedation of psychotropic drugs, a classification of drugs that affects the central nervous system.

The frequent use of hypnotic medications, such as sleep aids, can lead to a state of confusion or delirium. Clinical experience also suggests that in older persons short-acting psychotropics have longer-lasting effects, which replicate symptoms of dementia. However, the withdrawal of problematic drugs that affect the central nervous system has been shown to significantly improve cognitive function (Caird and Scott, 1986; Larson et al. 1987; Morrison and Katz 1989).

In order to assist clinicians in monitoring the side effects of drug interactions, family members and caregivers should be encouraged to keep a complete record of all the patient's medications, dosages, schedules of administration, as well as notations of any unusual reactions. This record should be brought with the patient to a healthcare provider.

A reminder that, for the purposes of recordkeeping, the terms "drugs" or "medications" include all OTC products including vitamins, supplements, and herbal remedies. People need to know that, as a courtesy, most pharmacies will keep a computerized record of medications prescribed by all their physicians.

It is imperative for all healthcare providers to consider the consequences medications that affect the central nervous system have on the elderly because they are commonly used by older adults and because the brain is the most vulnerable of human systems (Oslin 2000).

Alcoholism

Abuse of alcohol and legal drugs, both prescribed and over-the-counter, is a serious health problem among older Americans. This "invisible epidemic" affects about 15 percent of adults age sixty and older, a rapid-growth segment of America's population (SAMHSA 1998).

About 1 percent of all hospitalizations for elderly persons in the United States are due to alcoholism, yet the disorder remains an under-recognized problem among elderly primary care patients. Evidence exists that shows many primary care patients sixty years of age and older had current signs of alcoholism. However, fewer than half had alcohol abuse documented in their medical records. Older alcoholic patients were more likely than similar-aged nonalcoholic patients to be hospitalized and die, according to researchers (Ewing 1984).

Geriatric alcoholism is well hidden and can be an outgrowth of a chronic disorder or suddenly triggered by a life-altering change. Bereavement and retirement are two notable examples. Shifts in employment and death of friends or loved ones can activate loneliness, boredom, anxiety, and depression. In fact, alcohol misuse in older adults is linked with depression. The highest rate of new alcoholism is reported to be among elderly men who have lost their wives (Gambert 1997). These individuals are often able to avoid early detection because their drinking takes place at home and while alone.

Any use of drugs in combination with alcohol carries risk, and multiple drug abuse intensifies the hazards even more. Alcoholism can affect mental status, not only by its damage to hepatic (liver) function and the consumer's nutritional condition but also by direct toxic effects on the brain. Alcoholism is usually not suspected in elderly patients unless a lifelong problem has been noted. Increasingly, however, it is being seen as an issue among older people.

Alcohol merits special attention because the aging process affects how the body handles alcohol in late life. There is research suggesting that sensitivity to alcohol's health effects may increase with age (Dufour and Fuller 1995). One reason is that the older adult reaches a higher blood alcohol concentration (BAC) than younger people after consuming an equal amount of alcohol. The higher BAC results from an age-related decrease of body water in which to dilute the alcohol.

Alcohol is metabolized more slowly as a person ages and can cause alterations in cognition and perception of spaces and events, thereby increasing the risk for falls. Consuming alcohol in conjunction with medication can cause increased fatigue and confusion. Consequently, alcohol intake should be limited so as not to impair balance, coordination, and mental alertness.

Aging also interferes with the body's ability to tolerate alcohol. Therefore, elderly individuals persist in exhibiting certain effects of alcohol, primarily poor coordination, at lower amounts than younger adults whose tolerance *increases* with increased consumption.

Certain disorders, such as hypertension and diabetes, can worsen with alcohol use.

Many medications, prescriptions, OTC products, and herbal remedies can be dangerous, even deadly, when mixed with alcohol. This is a particular concern for seniors because most take multiple medications (Routledge, O'Mahony, and Woodhouse 2004).

As example, aspirin can cause bleeding in the stomach and intestines, a risk that is elevated if the individual is drinking alcohol. Cold and allergy medications—antihistamines—often cause drowsiness that is intensified when combined with alcohol. People who drink alcohol regularly are especially susceptible to acetaminophen-induced liver damage. Even drinking a small amount of alcohol can impair judgment, coordination, and reaction time. It can increase the risk of work and household accidents, including falls and hip fractures. These occurrences are often erroneously attributed to dementia.

> Some over-the-counter products such as cough syrups and laxatives have a high alcohol content.

Aging and alcoholism seem to produce some similar deficits in cognitive and behavioral functioning. Evidence shows alcoholism may accelerate normal aging or cause premature aging of the brain. When using magnetic resonance imaging (MRI) techniques, Dr. A. Pfefferbaum and colleagues found more brain tissue loss in subjects with alcoholism than in those without alcoholism, even after their ages had been taken into account. This occurred despite similar total life-time alcohol consumption. The results strongly suggested that aging increases the individual's susceptibility to alcohol's effects (Pfefferbaum et al. 1997).

Evidence also indicates that atrophy of the frontal lobes increases with alcohol consumption and is associated with intellectual impairment in both older and younger adults with alcoholism. Moreover, older alcoholics were found less likely to recover from cognitive deficits during abstinence than younger subjects (Volkow et al. 1997).

Alcohol can make some medical concerns hard for doctors to find and treat. For example, alcohol causes changes in the heart and blood vessels. These changes can dull pain that might be a warning sign of a heart attack. Drinking also can make older people forgetful and confused. These symptoms could be mistaken for signs of Alzheimer's disease. For people with diabetes, drinking affects blood sugar levels and makes them confused and lethargic, which may be mistaken for dementia.

Additionally, alcohol heightens the severity of certain medical conditions such as hypertension, ulcers, and diabetes. Alcoholism in the geriatric population is often overlooked when assessing an elderly individual for confusion or memory deficits.

The National Institute on Alcohol Abuse and Alcoholism, part of the National Institutes of Health, recommends that people over age sixty-five who choose to drink have no more than one drink a day. Drinking at this level usually is not associated with health risks.

Signs of Possible Alcohol Abuse

- Drinking to calm your nerves, forget your worries, or reduce depression
- Gulping down drinks
- Frequently having more than one drink a day; a standard drink is one 12-ounce bottle or can of beer or wine cooler, one 5-ounce glass of wine, or 1.5 ounces of 80-proof distilled spirits
- Lying about or trying to hide drinking habits
- Hurting yourself, or someone else, while drinking
- Feeling irritable, resentful, or unreasonable when not drinking
- Having medical, social, or financial worries caused by drinking

Source: National Institute on Alcohol Abuse and Alcoholism

Delirium

Delirium is not a disease; it is an acute state of confusion. The mental status changes in delirium develop over hours to days and represent a significant decline in the level of cognitive functioning. Since delirium should be considered a medical emergency and the manifestations of delirium are often confused with dementia, it is imperative that the patient be thoroughly evaluated before a diagnosis is made (Alagia-krishnan and Blanchette 2005).

Delirium is a temporary, usually reversible cause of cerebral dysfunction. The clinical hallmarks are anxiety, decreased attention span, hallucinations, delusions, and incoherence. The syndrome is often unrecognized or misdiagnosed. Commonly it is mistaken for depression, acute schizophrenic reaction, or just another element of old age.

DSM-IV Criteria for Delirium

- Disturbance of consciousness (reduced clarity of awareness of the environment) with reduced ability to focus, sustain, or shift attention
- A change in cognition (such as memory deficit, disorientation, language disturbance) or the development of a perceptual disturbance that is not better accounted for by a preexisting, established, or evolving dementia
- The disturbance develops over a short period of time (usually hours to days) and tends to fluctuate during the course of the day

Source: *Diagnostic and Statistical Manual of Mental Disorders,* fourth ed., 1995

Despite the fact that delirium is quite common in older persons with acute or chronic illnesses, it is not well recognized in clinical settings. In order to improve the clinical recognition of delirium, mental status tests need to be used to identify patients with cognitive impairment and establish the symptoms' history of onset and degree of fluctuations. Some of the underlying causes of delirium are infections, medications, metabolic and endocrine dysfunction, fecal impaction, urinary retention, and changes in the person's environment. Failure to diagnose delirium will have serious consequences.

Among the social and environmental factors that involve high levels of stress is a commonly overlooked trigger of altered mental status: hospital admission. Any frail, worried, elderly individual, thrust into a busy and unfamiliar hospital environment, surrounded by strangers, can quickly become confused and disoriented (Eriksson 1999).

If delirium is recognized early, it may be possible to prevent physical or mental disability and an irreversible deterioration. A person who displays the following symptoms is more likely to have delirium rather than uncomplicated dementia:

- Sudden onset of cognitive impairment
- Disorientation
- Disturbances in attention
- Decline in level of consciousness
- Perceptual disturbances (for example, hallucinations)

In addition to common medical conditions, any adverse effects of the following classifications of drugs are also common causes of delirium:

- Anticholinergic agents (used to treat a variety of conditions, from asthma and gastrointestinal cramps to motion sickness)
- Antipsychotic agents
- Antidepressants
- Digoxin
- H_2-blocking agents (drugs used to treat gastric reflux, heartburn, and indigestion)
- Antihypertensive agents

Depression

Depression is the most common of all mood or emotional disorders in the elderly, and it is often mistaken for Alzheimer's disease because elderly individuals display symptoms that are not as common. Typically an older depressed individual describes physical complaints, appears apathetic, and denies being depressed. Depression is more fully addressed in chapter 4.

Metabolic and Endocrine Disorders

Some of the prominent metabolic disorders associated with dementia are fluid and electrolyte imbalance, and liver and kidney disease. Calcium and sodium imbalances (either excesses or deficiencies) may cause confusion, personality changes, severe mental dysfunction, and dementia. When blood sugar or blood pressure is not maintained at normal or near normal levels, mental impairment often occurs.

Older adults are especially sensitive to dehydration, a condition that can be brought about by a short period of vomiting and diarrhea or exposure to summer heat with confusion and disorientation resulting. There are also certain drugs, particularly diuretics, that can cause confusion. Since brain cells are susceptible to dehydration, confusion is a reliable indicator that the dehydration has become severe.

Some common endocrine disorders are associated with altered mental status. The thyroid gland, for example, plays a key role in the body's metabolic function by controlling how the body burns energy, creates proteins, and moderates reactions among hormones. Thyroid disorders develop if the gland produces too much or too little of the amount of thyroid hormone required for healthy metabolic function. Hyperthyroidism results when there is excess production. Underproduction of thyroid hormone, or hypothyroidism, when left untreated can lead to physical and mental impairment with the resulting change in mental status often being mistaken for dementia.

Although age alone does not change the way the thyroid functions, some common disorders of the elderly make the diagnosis and treatment more challenging.

Other examples of such age-related metabolic and endocrine disorders are malnutrition, poorly controlled diabetes, and liver disease. Highlighting the gravity of thyroid disorders is the fact that 60 percent of older patients with hyperthyroidism have congestive heart failure. Other common findings are refractory atrial fibrillation (a condition where the upper chambers of the heart beat irregularly), weight loss, depression, lethargy, dementia, and confusion (Khaira and Franklyn 1999).

Sensory Deficits

Since the brain receives information by way of the senses, any sensory deficit sharply reduces an individual's ability to interpret information. There are people who are reluctant to admit they need hearing aids, and even when equipped with the appropriate devices, they often neglect to wear them. Lacking such assistive devices, though, means that the person cannot process information accurately and as a result may appear to an outside observer to be confused or cognitively impaired.

Nutritional Deficiencies

Vitamins are indispensable for a person's optimum health and well-being. Key parts of the brain may be damaged as a result of vitamin deficiencies, particularly a lack of B vitamins, which are essential for cell metabolism. Malnutrition is a common condition among elderly individuals and this situation places them at risk for a vitamin B_{12} deficiency, one of the most common nutritional causes of reversible dementia (Bottiglieri 1996).

Symptoms of a B_{12} deficiency are difficulty in maintaining balance, depression, confusion, and poor memory. This emphasizes again the importance of ruling out other contributing possibilities before a positive diagnosis of an irreversible dementia is made.

Up to 30 percent of adults fifty years and older may have atrophic gastritis, an overgrowth of intestinal flora, benign microorganisms that normally live in the gastrointestinal tract and are essential for digestion. They may also be unable to normally absorb vitamin B_{12} in food. However, they are able to absorb the synthetic B_{12} added to fortified foods and dietary supplements. Vitamin supplements and fortified foods may be the best sources of vitamin B_{12} for adults over the age of fifty. Scientists have long been interested in the potential connection between vitamin B_{12} deficiency and dementia (Eastley, Wilcock, and Bucks 2000). The research suggests vitamin B_{12} deficiency may decrease levels of substances needed for the metabolism of neurotransmitters, chemicals that transmit nerve signals. Consequently, the reduced levels of neurotransmitters may result in cognitive impairment (Hutto 1997).

Taking vitamin B_{12} is virtually without risk. The Institute of Medicine (IOM) of the National Academy of Sciences has no established Tolerable Upper Intake Level for this vitamin because it has a very low potential for toxicity. Up to 30 percent of those individuals over the age of fifty years, regardless of the type of diet they follow, lose their ability to digest the protein-bound form of the vitamin that is present in eggs, dairy, and other animal products, thus *all* people over the age of fifty should use vitamin B_{12} supplements or fortified foods. The Institute of Medicine maintains that "no adverse effects have been associated with excess vitamin B_{12} intake from food and supplements in healthy individuals." People who follow a vegan diet, which excludes not only meat but also eggs and milk, may also require supplementary vitamin B_{12} (IOM 1998).

Individuals who drink excessive amounts of alcohol over a long period of time sometimes develop a deficiency of vitamin B1 (thiamine). This deficiency leads to the mental and physical problems that are often seen in chronic alcoholics. Inadequate B_{12} may be due to nutritional deficiencies, malabsorption syndromes, or a variety of gastrointestinal causes.

Normal Pressure Hydrocephalus

Normal pressure hydrocephalus (NPH) is a brain disorder that develops gradually over a period of time when the flow of cerebrospinal fluid (CSF) is blocked. The fluid fills up within the spaces in the brain, which in turn compresses brain tissue. The affected person may lose any or all brain functions controlled by the area of the brain that is affected.

Risk factors include disorders that may cause obstruction of the flow of CSF, such as closed head injury, brain surgery, an infection (meningitis, for example), and bleeding from a blood vessel or aneurysm in the brain. In most cases, however, the cause is unknown. When NPH is successfully treated, the associated dementia generally is reversed. It is thought to account for about 5 percent of all dementias (Verrees and Selman 2004).

Infections

As a rule, most people are unaware of how threatening infections can be to older adults. Since their symptoms are often found to be atypical, they can be difficult to diagnose. Two of the most common causes of a missed diagnosis are the absence of a fever and receiving normal results from laboratory tests. A frequent finding is that a change in mental status or a decline in function may be the only problem present in an older patient with an infection.

An estimated 90 percent of deaths resulting from pneumonia occur in people sixty-five years and older. Mortality resulting from influenza also occurs primarily in the elderly. The diagnosis of pneumonia in older adults is difficult to make since the signs and symptoms can be understated. Consequently, the initiation of antibiotic therapy is often delayed, which may contribute to higher mortality rates (Crossley and Peterson 1998).

Urinary tract infections (UTIs) are the most frequent bacterial infection and the most common source of bacteremia (bacteria in the blood) in older adults. Older adults are predisposed to UTIs when catheters are used or if they have developed neurogenic bladders with increased residual urine (McCue 1999).

Neurogenic bladder is the loss of normal bladder function caused by damage to part of the nervous system. The damage can cause the bladder to become underactive, meaning it is unable to contract and empty completely, or it can be overactive and contract too quickly or frequently.

Factors that contribute to neurogenic bladder include prostate enlargement in men and vaginal atrophy in women. Along with vaginal atrophy, there is a concurrent incomplete emptying of the bladder in women. These features provide the opportunity for bacterial colonization and are likely to contribute to the higher rates of asymptomatic bacteriuria (an increased amount of bacteria in urine, which causes increased frequency of urination and burning) and UTIs in the elderly (Zhanel, Harding, and Guay 1990).

Dementia, as evidenced by lethargy, agitation, and other changes in mental status, is often the primary signal of both pneumonia and urinary tract infections.

Arteriosclerosis

Ateriosclerosis, popularly called "hardening of the arteries," is used to describe several diseases that involve the heart and blood vessels, components of the cardiovascular system. Veins and arteries that thicken and lose their elasticity are unable to supply sufficient blood to the brain, thus causing damage to brain cells, followed by small strokes or infarcts. Multi-infarct dementia (see p. 22), a type of vascular dementia, is often the end result.

It is always a challenge for clinicians to differentiate between reversible and irreversible dementias since the symptoms can be caused by a large number of underlying physical disorders that have the capability of affecting brain function in the elderly. The symptoms of individuals who are experiencing depression or drug toxicity may be very similar to the symptoms of patients with early-stage Alzheimer's disease or a vascular dementia. There is a range of treatments for those illnesses and the outcomes differ markedly.

HYPERTENSION AND THE LINK TO DEMENTIA

It is well known that hypertension, for example, chronic high blood pressure, can cause a stroke or brain attack, which will damage the brain. Hypertension is a serious problem affecting the global population. This disorder is pervasive with an estimated 600 million people worldwide suffering with the disease. One of the main concerns is the fact that millions of people are unaware that they are hypertensive, since the disease has no overt symptoms. This is why it is referred to as a "silent" disease. However, it is a health problem that no one can afford to ignore, since high blood pressure greatly increases a person's risk of heart disease and stroke (Mensah 2004).

Blood pressure is determined by the amount of blood pumped by the heart, and the size and condition of the arteries. Many other factors can affect blood pressure, including volume of water in the body; salt content of the body; condition of the kidneys, nervous system, or blood vessels; and levels of various hormones in the body.

Essential hypertension has no identifiable cause. It may be caused by genetics, environmental factors, and dietary elements such as salt consumption. Secondary hypertension is high blood pressure caused by another disorder. Among the many contributing maladies are adrenal gland tumors, kidney disorders, oral contraceptives, drugs, or other chemicals.

A broad collection of research studies reflect a range of lifestyle elements, including diet and nutrition, cholesterol levels, body weight, exercise, and blood pressure, all of which when kept within normal limits have a role in preventing or delaying the onset of Alzheimer's disease and vascular dementia. The Ninth International Conference on Alzheimer's Disease and Related Disorders (ICAD) in Philadelphia 2004 presented evidence suggesting that the same factors putting us at risk for heart attacks also put us at risk for dementia.

A recent long-term study of fifteen hundred middle-aged and elderly Finns revealed that the link between cardiovascular disease and dementia has become more pronounced in recent years. People who exercised in middle age were found to be far less likely to develop AD and other types of dementia. This was the first study to illustrate the long-term association between physical activity and dementia later in life. Specifically, the findings showed that middle-aged people who exercised at least twice a week had a 50 percent lower chance of developing dementia and a 60 percent lower chance of developing AD than their sedentary peers (Kivipelto 2005).

Since vascular disease and dementia appear to be related, consumers as well as health professionals need to understand that what is good for the heart is good for the brain. Following a heart healthy diet and increasing physical activity seems to be a strong defense against developing dementia.

Hypertension may be indicated when blood pressure is high at any single measurement. Hypertension is confirmed through repeated blood pressure measurements over time. Blood pressure that is consistently 140 or higher systolic (measures the pressure of the blood when the heart contracts and pushes blood through the circulatory system), or 90 or higher diastolic (measures the pressure of the blood when the heart relaxes between contractions), indicates hypertension. Both numbers, systolic and diastolic, are equally important and the elevation of either number will indicate hypertension.

Measurement guidelines for diagnosing and monitoring hypertension are:

- Prehypertension: systolic pressure consistently 120 to 139, or diastolic 80 to 89
- Stage 1 hypertension: systolic pressure consistently 140 to 159, or diastolic 90 to 99
- Stage 2 hypertension: systolic pressure consistently 160 or over, or diastolic 100 or over

High blood pressure is more likely to develop if an individual has prehypertension. Typically, however, lifestyle changes such as not smoking, weight loss, moderation of alcohol intake, adequate exercise, and a healthy diet can prevent this. Even small improvements can result in very rewarding gains for people at risk.

Untreated chronic hypertension can lead to stroke, blood vessel damage, heart attack, and heart and kidney failure. Before initiating treatment clinicians require blood tests to assess organ and tissue damage and other risk factors. These tests include electrocardiogram, urinalysis, blood cell count, and blood chemistry, which consists of measuring levels of potassium, sodium, creatinine, fasting glucose, total and high-density lipoprotein (HDL) cholesterol, or the "good" cholesterol. Any additional tests will be recommended based on the physician's findings.

Dementia causes a high burden of suffering for patients, their families, and society. However, according to some studies, more than half of people with dementia have never been diagnosed (O'Connor et al. 1988; Valcour et al. 2000). There are many conditions that cause dementia. If the cause is treatable, the dementia may be dramatically reversed. It is therefore vitally important to the patient that a thorough medical assessment be made so an appropriate treatment plan can be devised and implemented.

Chapter 2

Mild Cognitive Impairment

An Early Warning?

The strongest risk factor for dementia is age, and the risk of dementia in older adults increases with each decade. An estimated 11 percent of individuals sixty-five years of age and older, and nearly half of those eighty-five years of age and older, have dementia (Bodarty et al. 2000).

A question that has intrigued researchers for many years is why some people remain cognitively healthy all their lives while others develop dementia. For example, there are elderly individuals who always maintain very high cognitive performance levels. They never seem to lose their "edge." Other seniors experience a decline in certain cognitive abilities that seems to coincide with a number of common weaknesses in their physical condition. There is also a third group that develops memory problems to a much greater degree than is expected for their age. However, these memory problems do not necessarily meet all the accepted criteria for Alzheimer's disease (AD). These people may have a condition called mild cognitive impairment (MCI).

Mild cognitive impairment is characterized by an impaired memory for someone who functions normally in all other cognitive areas. Scientists further describe it as a transition between changes in the brain due to normal aging and the more serious impairments caused by AD (Petersen et al. 1999). The disorder is distinguished solely by trouble with remembering. Researchers investigate it as a brain illness in which a person's memory processes and the related nerve cells gradually deteriorate prior to a slow descent into AD, the most common form of dementia. The results of the more recent research indicate that the rate of mild cognitive impairment in persons age seventy-five and older is higher than expected, affecting approximately 22 percent of the elderly (Lopez et al. 2003).

Mild cognitive impairment is not the same as the normal memory changes due to aging. Most unimpaired older adults have momentary lapses, such as misplacing something, or forgetting a friend's name or where they parked the car. Memory loss associated with MCI, however, is more persistent and troublesome. Elders with MCI have significantly more difficulty remembering information after a rather short period of time has elapsed. For example, when tested for research purposes, certain subjects remembered much less of a paragraph they read or details of simple drawings they saw compared to people with the usual age-related memory changes. Studies have also found, though, that many people with mild cognitive impairment do not progress to dementia and some even revert to normal cognitive functioning. This has led researchers to conclude MCI may be far more varied than once was thought and also the condition represents more than just a precursor to AD (Ganguli et al. 2004).

CRITERIA FOR DIAGNOSIS: SIGNS AND SYMPTOMS

In 2001 the American Academy of Neurology (AAN) published practice guidelines for the early detection of memory problems. The following criteria were identified by the academy for a diagnosis as mild cognitive impairment.

- An individual's report of his or her own memory problems, preferably confirmed by another person
- Measurable, greater-than-normal memory impairment, detected with standard assessment tests
- Normal overall thinking and reasoning skills
- Ability to perform normal daily activities
- Absence of dementia

The criteria, however, also raised more questions about the subtle yet measurable memory disorder.

Over the years there has been rising interest in researching the significant increase of mild intellectual deterioration that is seen in many elderly individuals. Studies often refer to isolated memory impairment, incipient dementia, benign senescent forgetfulness, or age-associated cognitive decline. Many changes in brain function have been measured in the elderly and are due to the normal physiologic changes of aging through the years. These include slower rates of learning and remembering new information; less efficient working memory (or information needed for a short time, such as parking location after shopping); declines in language ability (for example, incorrect spelling, sluggish retrieval of nouns); and increased difficulty performing several tasks at once (such as talking on the phone and working on the computer) (Voit 2002). A report from a Mayo Clinic study suggests that about 12 percent of those over seventy have MCI. Furthermore, those with the disorder are three to four times more likely to develop AD than those without such impairment.

MCI emerges in some individuals as a faulty memory that, although not as prominent as dementia, is more noticeable than the expected age-associated memory changes. It is important to remember, though, that while most people with this condition eventually develop dementia, some do not.

Memory skills are important to general cognitive functioning and low cognitive functioning (namely, memory impairment) is a major risk factor for nursing home placement. The risk for cognitive impairment is known to increase with age. Scientists have learned that as people age, the complex cognitive behaviors of attention, language, learning, and memory become exposed to injury and impairment. For many older adults this can result in declines in performance of everyday tasks such as driving or managing finances, which, in turn, causes worry and frustration. Eventually the situation leads to isolation from friends, loved ones, and society. At their worst, the problems that were first viewed as normal changes due to aging can become severe enough to be classified as MCI and, ultimately, as AD.

While people with MCI may have ongoing memory problems, by and large they are not plagued with the language and awareness deficits regularly seen in AD. Nor are they confused. Generally such individuals seem to have memory problems greater than those usually expected in the elderly, yet not as severe as the other, more troubling symptoms characteristic of AD, especially when it involves accomplishing their daily activities.

Ordinarily, people suspected of having MCI still retain their personalities and social skills. Although they may remember very few current events, details of recent conversations, or names of people they just met, initially their memory problems do not seem to be serious. MCI is difficult to diagnose because, although the evidence may point to a brain disorder, the clinician also needs to evaluate the many interacting common age-related changes.

IDENTIFYING MILD COGNITIVE IMPAIRMENT (MCI)

In the early stages of dementia, when the physician is attempting to make a first diagnosis, the patient may demonstrate different levels of cognitive and functional competence. Some examples are driving without getting lost or taking medications without difficulty but then forgetting three-fourths of the items in a delayed-recall task. Scientists are developing additional ways to identify individuals who are suspected of having MCI. In particular, they are studying those older adults who demonstrate memory loss but who do not meet the established criteria for a diagnosis of AD. Imaging studies of people with MCI have yielded helpful information when compared with unaffected people of similar age and health status. The researchers found that the smaller the hippocampus (a region of the brain associated with learning and memory) and the more rapidly it shrinks during the aging process, the more likely an individual is to become cognitively impaired (Blalock et al. 2003). Newer research, however, also suggests that there are other ways to identify people at risk of AD, even before MCI develops (Prichep 2005).

Currently, what is known is that older adults with MCI already have:

- A significant decrease in the number of neurons (nerve cells) in the brain
- A reduction in the volume of an important memory center in the brain called the entorhinal cortex, the threshold to a neighboring area of the brain important for learning and memory called the hippocampus
- Reduction in the size of the hippocampus, which is one of the areas first affected by AD

These alterations are associated with very early cognitive changes and strongly suggest that brain damage due to MCI or AD may start a long time before the disease is diagnosed (Petersen 2001).

Scientists have defined subtypes of MCI based on cause, for example, degenerative, vascular, psychiatric (especially depression), and medical, and based on which aspects of cognition are most affected. The subtype that is characterized chiefly by memory impairment is called MCI with memory loss, or amnestic mild cognitive impairment. It is this subtype that is most likely to lead to AD.

Individuals with other MCI subtypes may have prominent deficits in other cognitive functions, such as language skills or visuospatial ability. These types of dementia can be caused by other degenerative diseases, for example, frontotemporal dementia, dementia with Lewy bodies, or vascular dementia (Petersen 2004).

> At the World Alzheimer Congress 2000, held in Washington, DC, it was revealed that there has been significant progress in distinguishing individuals with benign memory difficulties from those with the onset of AD.

NORMAL BRAIN AGING, MILD COGNITIVE IMPAIRMENT, AND ALZHEIMER'S DISEASE

During the aging process many normal changes occur throughout the body, including in the brain. The shrinkage of neurons is commonplace in this highly specialized organ that governs, among many diverse functions, our thinking, reasoning, and emotions. (This change is particularly evident in areas of the brain that regulate and control memory, learning, planning, and other complex mental activities.)

Essentially, the alterations cause a slower processing of information that, in turn, affects recall ability and other brain functions. The course of events is termed *age-associated cognitive decline*. Nevertheless, all the systems of the brain are not affected equally and in some older individuals the changes are barely noticeable.

Other normal physiologic changes in the brain that are natural products of aging are

- The development of amyloid plaques and neurofibrillary tangles although in smaller amounts than what is seen in AD
- Increased inflammation of brain tissue
- Increased damage caused by free radicals, which are highly reactive molecules that readily combine with other molecules. These can be produced from inside the body, or be introduced externally by pollutants and toxins, from smoking, for example.

Nerve cells become damaged when accumulation of these molecules is excessive.

Healthy older adults notice these changes when they find that learning new information or retrieving some data from the past takes longer than it used to. Although the deficits may be frustrating at times, there is no interference with the ability to perform daily activities.

A NEW LOOK AT NORMAL BRAIN AGING

In the past, significant loss in the ability to remember, learn, think, and reason, the skills known collectively as cognition, was considered a normal part of aging. Research shows that most people remain both relatively alert and mentally able as they age, and that severe cognitive loss is the result of disease. Dementia is suspected when a person experiences a substantial decline in memory as well as other changes in cognition, personality, or both.

There is increased attention being focused on research of normal brain aging. Current evidence indicates that as a person ages, most regions of the brain remain structurally sound. Contrary to what was once thought, there is no general widespread loss of brain neurons as people grow old. "Although there is some loss, it's far less than once believed and appears to be confined to certain highly select areas, with those areas essential for memory largely spared," states Dr. Guy McKhann, professor of neurology and neuroscience at Johns Hopkins and director of the School of Medicine's Zanvyl Krieger Mind/Brain Institute (McKhann and Albert 2002).

Furthermore, there are parts of the brain, such as the hippocampus, where new nerve cells are formed well into old age. Nonetheless, there is increasing evidence that over time, noticeable cellular and molecular changes take place in the brain (Stadtman 1992; Merck 2000). These physical modifications are responsible for many changes in brain-related functions that have been measured in older adults, such as nondementia memory loss and cognitive declines; "tip-of-the-tongue" problems; impairments in vision, hearing, and taste; and changes in sleep rhythms and sleep quality.

As people age, their memories for recent events tend to become less precise, less well specified (Glisky, Rubin, and Davidson 2001). Healthy older people typically have attention deficits as well. The inability of most older people to ignore distractions is the main reason why memory problems abound in seniors. "Difficulty filtering out distractions impacts a wide range of daily life activities such as driving, social interactions and reading, and can greatly affect quality of life," writes Dr. Adam Gazzaley, lead researcher in a study on aging and memory at the University of California, Berkeley (Gazzaley 2005).

There are individuals who develop cognitive and memory problems that are not severe enough to be diagnosed as dementia but are more pronounced than the cognitive changes associated with normal aging. As an example, there are countless elders with obvious memory impairments who function in other areas such as making decisions, calling family members and friends by name, and caring for their own basic needs. These individuals exhibit isolated memory complaints

Figure 2.1. Signs of Normal Cognitive Decline Compared with MCI

Normal Cognitive Decline	Mild Cognitive Impairment
Slower rates of learning	Ongoing memory problems
Less ability to retain information	Normal judgment, reasoning skills
Decline in language skills; for example, in spelling, sluggish noun retrieval	Able to complete activities of daily living
Difficulty multitasking	Absence of dementia

with their daily activities, but they lack cognitive deficits in certain areas that are required for a diagnosis of AD. These are the people who are categorized as having MCI. Although many of them will go on to develop AD, at this time it is unclear that a progression to AD is inevitable.

Here are some recommended behavioral and social activities essential for good health and function that can help to protect and improve the mental abilities of older adults.

- Make a habit of exercising regularly. Regular exercise can assist in the treatment and prevention of many diseases affecting older adults—such as diabetes, hypertension, coronary artery disease, osteoporosis, colon cancer, obesity, and depression (Zagaria 2002). Walking twenty to thirty minutes three or four times a week is associated with improved cardiac function, maintenance of muscle strength, and reduced risk of osteoporosis.
- Reading, learning a new skill, and playing board games or *any* game in which planning and devising strategies are involved.
- Strengthen social contacts by cultivating relationships with family and friends. Consider volunteering. (Contact a senior services agency for more information.)
- Fortify resistance to disease by improving nutrition through the increase in consumption of fruits, vegetables, and whole grains, and the decrease of fat and sugar intake. Other positive steps are getting the influenza and pneumococcal vaccines as advised, maintaining appropriate blood sugar and cholesterol levels, and keeping weight and blood pressure at normal levels. Be more attentive to hand washing.

WHY IS MILD COGNITIVE IMPAIRMENT CONTROVERSIAL?

Currently most clinicians view mild cognitive impairment as a risk or transition stage for the development of Alzheimer's disease. However, the term is nonspecific and as such it promotes an indecisive general-ization of late-life dementia. This ambiguity helps to perpetuate the conventional view of elders as being frail and confused, unable to learn anything new, and in need of supervision. As a result, the true significance of memory problems is obscured, and valuable time that could be spent evaluating a cognitively impaired patient is lost.

The development of MCI, for example, is strongly associated with depression and cerebrovascular disease (Lopez et al. 2003). Moreover, it is well known by healthcare professionals that both depression and cerebrovascular disease can be treated. Cardiorespiratory fitness, which includes activities such as bicycling, swimming, and walking, is also associated with the preservation of overall cognitive function and attention in healthy older adults (Barnes 2003; Newson and Kemps 2006).

There are more potentially important benefits of early detection, including:

- Providing the chance for individuals and their caregivers to plan ahead
- Discussing treatment strategies
- Developing social support
- Adapting living arrangements
- Making a will, assigning power of attorney, designating a healthcare proxy (Patterson and Gass 2001)

MCI is a comparatively recent diagnostic description that is still ques-tioned by many in the medical community. No completely reliable means, other than long-term follow-up and eventual autopsy, exists yet to distinguish between patients experiencing MCI due to preclin-ical AD and patients experiencing MCI due to less frequently occur-ring conditions (Petersen et al. 2001).

Although memory loss (amnestic MCI) is the chief complaint, reaching a diagnosis is further complicated by the strong likelihood of sensory losses, namely, vision and hearing deficits that are widespread in the geriatric population (Morris and Cummings 2005). Additionally, it is seldom possible to confirm how long any of the symptoms have existed in a person before medical attention is sought.

Another barrier to the identification and treatment of mild cognitive impairment is that it illustrates one of the more prominent myths about aging firmly held by some health professionals and a great proportion of the general public, namely, that substantial memory loss among the elderly is normal. Until this dilemma is successfully resolved, the long lag time between the appearance of symptoms and a medical assessment followed by therapeutic intervention will persist.

Although most older adults exhibit minimal decrease in cognitive function, research suggests that nearly 10 percent of all people over age sixty-five and up to half of those over age eighty-five have AD or another dementia. As the population of older Americans increases, so will the number of people with AD (AAGP 2004).

When a cognitive impairment is found in an older person, it may reflect a number of conditions, many of them reversible. Some of the possibilities to be considered include:

- Effects of medication
- Late-life depression
- Endocrine disorders
- Stroke
- Normal pressure hydrocephalus
- Alcoholism

Individuals who are only mildly impaired can be quite adept at concealing what is happening to them. And all too often family members quickly shrug off their loved one's memory impairment by attributing it to old age, stress, or general absentmindedness. However, most primary care physicians can, through standard testing and private interviewing (to ensure that a family member cannot prompt the patient), diagnose and treat most persistent or worsening cognitive problems.

Since there are multiple causes of forgetting, there is no standard explanation as to why a person has a faulty memory. The critical first step is to determine the cause by having a professional clinical evaluation. Once the cause is determined, both patient and family can learn what to do about the problem.

THE TWO MOST COMMON CAUSES OF COGNITIVE IMPAIRMENT IN OLDER ADULTS

Two of the most common causes of reversible dementia are adverse drug reactions and depression. Elderly individuals are more likely than younger patients to develop a cognitive impairment as a result of taking a medication. This reflects age and illness-associated changes in brain neurochemistry and changes in organ function and drug metabolism. Delirium, an acute confusional state, is the cognitive disturbance most clearly associated with drug toxicity, but dementia has also been reported. Drug-induced confusion can be prevented by avoiding taking of multiple drugs at the same time and adhering to the saying "start low and go slow" (Moore and O'Keeffe 1999).

There is a stigma associated with depression, and patients often try to hide the symptoms. However, there is sufficient evidence indicating the possibility that depression is a risk factor for dementia and cognitive decline (Jorm 2000).

The practice of taking multiple medications concurrently—polypharmacy—plays a key role in adverse drug reactions. Elders generally tend to have more long-term, chronic illnesses such as hypertension, diabetes, arthritis, and cardiovascular disease than younger people. As a result, people ages sixty-five and older consume more prescription and over-the-counter medicines than any other age group. Older Americans spend an average total of $3 billion annually on prescription medications (Heinrich 2001). These consumers buy 30 percent of all prescription drugs and 40 percent of all OTC drugs. (The average elderly person takes approximately four prescribed medications daily plus two OTC drugs.) In fact, one study examined the medication habits of people aged eighty-five and older and estimated that the elderly may even use twice as many OTC medications as prescription medications (Conn 1992).

The use of herbs and other supplements is another practice that is quite common among seniors. Older individuals who use complementary and alternative medicine (CAM) often fail to mention it to their physicians, and physicians may overlook asking about their use. These factors quickly elevate the risk for elders who are taking numerous medications without knowledge of their combined effects. In light of their age-related decline in drug metabolism, older consumers are much more vulnerable than most to adverse interactions between their prescribed medications and any herbal remedies they use (Raji 2005). This is borne out by the number of visits to physicians' offices, hospital outpatient departments, and hospital emergency departments for adverse drug effects that are consistently higher in older adults than in children or younger adults (Zhan et al. 2005).

THE NATIONAL CENTER FOR COMPLEMENTARY AND ALTERNATIVE MEDICINE (NCCAM)

General and Health Information

Information specialists at the NCCAM Clearinghouse can answer questions about the center and complementary and alternative medicine.

Toll free: 1-888-644-6226
International: 301-519-3153
TTY (for hearing impaired): 1-866-464-3615
Fax: 1-866-464-3616
http://www.nccam.nih.gov

Adverse Drug Reactions

When two or more drugs are mixed in the body, they may interact and produce distressing or even dangerous side effects. It follows, then, that of all the problems older people face because of their medication use, drug interactions are probably the most risky (FDA 2003).

It is obvious that today's senior population benefits greatly from prescription drugs. However, drug treatment has become much more complex over the past few decades. New drugs become available every year, and new uses are found for existing drugs. Medicines now manage many of the diseases that at one time disabled people. However, these benefits generally come with risks and the consequences of drug misuse or drug interactions can be serious.

Before prescribing any new drug to an older patient, the clinician needs to be aware of *all* the drugs the patient may be taking. "Too often, older people get more drugs without a reassessment of their previous medications," says Madeline Feinberg, PharmD, a pharmacist and former director of the Elder Health Program of the University of Maryland School of Pharmacy.

In order to be effective, drugs go through four processes in the body. Initially they are absorbed, then distributed, metabolized, and eliminated. Certain physical changes caused by the aging process can affect any or all of these factors. As examples, lean body mass and fluid levels decrease with age while fat reserves increase. These alterations affect drug distribution. The decline in liver and kidney function affects drug metabolism and elimination. These bodily changes associated with aging can change what constitutes the appropriate dosage for any particular person. When age-related changes decrease absorption or distribution of the drug, a higher dosage may be needed. On the other hand, age-related changes that decrease drug metabolism and elimination may mean that a lower dosage may achieve the same effect. Generally, for elders, these changes mean that medications take longer to clear out of their systems than they do in middle-aged individuals (AGS 2005).

The first system to break down when the drug burden becomes too great is the nervous system. When dealing with confused elderly patients, many experienced physicians may simply try to eliminate all but the most essential drugs for a trial period. Often that is sufficient to clear the confusion. When a medication is reintroduced, the patients frequently are able to manage on far fewer drugs (McKhann et al. 1984).

Other common barriers to the safe and successful use of medication include:

- Not understanding the instructions because English is not the patient's first language
- Misunderstanding a physician or pharmacist because of hearing deficits
- Becoming alarmed by friends or family when told of someone else's adverse event
- Difficulty in budgeting for medications

There are additional issues regularly associated with medication-related problems. Some of the more frequently occurring examples are:

- Unnecessary drugs are prescribed
- The need for new or additional medications is overlooked
- The wrong medication is prescribed
- A prescribed dose is too low or too high
- The patient does not report known allergies
- The patient is noncompliant (for example, she fails to fill the prescription or take the drugs properly)

Noncompliance with drug therapy in older patient populations ranges from 21 to 55 percent (Botelho and Dudrak 1992; Coons et al. 1994; Billups et al. 2000).

Some patients may intentionally take too much of a medication, thinking it will help speed their recovery. They reason that "if two pills are good, four pills must be twice as good." There are individuals who cannot afford the medications or who may undermedicate in order to make their prescriptions last longer. A common and long-standing issue is that of patients who do not take a medication as prescribed. Noncompliance turns out to be more costly and more serious than a number of major illnesses.

One of the first steps in addressing noncompliance is to thoroughly understand the patient's perspective on the disease in question. Only then will simple interventions by the healthcare team, such as reinforcing the importance of taking the prescribed dose and encouraging use of pill calendars, boxes, and other types of dispensers, help to improve adherence and overall compliance with drug therapy (Kane, Ouslander, and Abrass 1999).

Steps That Help Reduce Polypharmacy

1. Have patients "brown bag" all medications at each office visit and keep an accurate record of all medications, including over-the-counter medications and herbs.
2. Know the side effects of the drugs being prescribed.
3. Be sure there is a medical need for the drug being prescribed.
4. Stop providing any drug to the patient that has no known benefit.
5. Stop providing any drug that is not clinically indicated.

Source: Williams 2002

Depression in Older Adults

It can be hard to tell the difference between late-life depression and a disorder such as dementia. Many of the symptoms are similar, such as having trouble recalling something, concentrating, or making decisions. Furthermore, older adults may be reluctant to talk to their doctor about sad or anxious feelings because they are embarrassed. But no one should be embarrassed by depression. It is not a personal weakness. Although depression is a serious and debilitating illness, it can be treated. (See chapter 4.)

TREATMENT FOR MILD COGNITIVE IMPAIRMENT

Individuals who are diagnosed with MCI may have significant differences in symptoms since there is no unanimity about a definition. Suggestions and recommendations for treatment may also vary. In most cases, however, clinicians will evaluate the patient periodically for changes in memory and thinking skills that suggest a worsening of symptoms or a progression to mild dementia (Petersen et al. 2001).

Recent findings have shown there is insufficient evidence to recommend for or against routine screening for dementia in asymptomatic older adults. However, the researchers also uncovered "good evidence that some screening tests have good sensitivity but, unfortunately, only fair specificity in detecting cognitive impairment and dementia." They also judged that some drug therapies have a beneficial effect on cognitive function (Boustani et al. 2003).

According to a presentation of preliminary data from a recently completed clinical trial supported by the National Institute on Aging, people with mild cognitive impairment who were taking the drug donepezil were at a lower risk of progressing to AD for the first eighteen months of a three-year study when compared with their counterparts who were given a placebo. But the reduced risk of progressing from MCI to AD among participants on donepezil disappeared after eighteen months; by the end of the study the likelihood of progressing to AD was the same in both groups (NIA 2004). During the study, patients with MCI were given donepezil, vitamin E, or a placebo. In addition to being tested for AD, the participants were evaluated in other, more specific areas of their cognitive function, for example, language, orientation, attention, and ability to perform their everyday activities. Although researchers found a lesser risk for AD with donepezil therapy, the effect appears to be short term. Nevertheless, researchers are optimistic that what was learned might allow better trials to be designed that could result in more effective treatment. The researchers said there was no apparent benefit from vitamin E.

This large clinical trial is the first to show that a drug can temporarily reduce the risk of transition to a clinical diagnosis of AD for some individuals with MCI.

IS ROUTINE SCREENING OF ALL ELDERLY DESIRABLE?

Most clinicians agree that routine mental status screening of all elderly individuals is probably not necessary. Such a practice would be expensive and impractical. Nonetheless, both the American Medical Association and the American Academy of Family Physicians urge clinicians to remain watchful for signs of cognitive or functional decline in their elderly patients that may signal the initial stages of dementia (Grace and Amick 2005).

There are several sound and compelling reasons why early recognition of cognitive impairment is so important:

- Diagnosis may uncover a potentially reversible medical situation
- Clinicians gain a valuable opportunity for timely treatment interventions
- Clinicians have more time to monitor the patient for compliance to medical recommendations
- Patients and caregivers gain time to plan for future lifestyle

changes, for example, financial arrangements and end-of-life care (Boutsani et al. 2003)

UNDERUTILIZATION OF THERAPIES

In normal aging, some of the important aspects of mental health include stable intellectual functioning and the capacity for change. With aging come certain alterations in mental functioning, but very few of these changes match the many pervasive and commonly held stereotypes about aging (Cohen and Herbert 1996; Rowe and Kahn 1997).

MCI is a health problem that may not receive clinical attention for a long time. As many as two-thirds of all cases of dementia in the community are neither recognized nor evaluated. According to Dr. P. Murali Doraiswamy, director of clinical trials in the Department of Psychiatry and Behavioral Sciences at Duke University, geriatric psychiatry specialists "haven't yet convinced primary care physicians of the value of treatment for dementia and cognitive disorders associated with AD. They thus have no real impctus to diagnose the disorder. The result is a large number of last-minute diagnoses that even a grocery store clerk could have made."

The mental health of older Americans is an important determinant of overall national well-being. Key indicators of well-being are measures drawn from the most reliable official statistics (Wallman 2004) and they illustrate both the promises and the difficulties that confront the elderly in the United States.

Recent research determined that not only is MCI prevalent in the elderly but also that most of the cognitive difficulties the affected individuals have can be traced to a variety of problems. Some examples are small "silent" brain lesions, depression, use of psychiatric medications, and other disease processes that can affect the brain. This emphasizes the importance of good medical care in preventing the development of brain disease (Lopez et al. 2003).

Dementia is suspected when a person experiences a substantial decline in memory as well as other changes in cognition, personality, or both. There is evidence suggesting that although there are few differences in the numbers or types of coexisting medical illnesses between individuals with MCI and those with dementia, the dementia patients are prescribed more medications (Lyketsos 2005). Nevertheless, the gravity of the coexisting illnesses is primarily associated with declines in day-to-day functioning and cognition. In the December 2001 *Archives of Neurology*, a team of specialists recommended further research to define subcategories of MCI. For example, a problem primarily with language rather than memory might be considered a type of MCI that is an early sign of a dementia other than AD (Petersen et al. 2001).

Future investigations need to explore the role of multiple illnesses and their treatment at the beginning or during development of dementia. Other key questions are:

- How much memory impairment is too much to be considered abnormal?
- How much memory impairment is significant enough to be considered a symptom of mild dementia?
- How hard should one look for subtle abnormalities in other areas of thinking?
- How do we know if these other changes are due to normal aging or dementia?

These unresolved issues about MCI give emphasis to the need for continuing research. The more pressing issue for families, however, is to lose no time looking into the reason for a loved one's impaired memory. The place to start is with the individual's primary care physician.

Chapter 3

Alzheimer's Disease

Going, Going, Gone!

There are now more than 5 million people in the United States living with Alzheimer's disease. This number includes 4.9 million people over the age of sixty-five and between 200,000 and 500,000 people under age sixty-five with early-onset Alzheimer's disease and other dementias (AA 2007).

The number of older adults in the United States and other developed countries is unprecedented and is still growing. It is a phenomenon that has prompted researchers to focus their efforts on the effects aging has on health. The trend is timely as well as practical since one of the most feared consequences of growing older is Alzheimer's disease (AD).

The development of AD can best be compared to a series of thefts. AD slowly and inexorably robs a person of his memory, intellect, and all physical abilities. However, patients are not the only casualties of the disease. As AD advances over time, individuals who were once vigorous and self-reliant become frail and totally dependent on overwhelmed caregivers for all of their most basic needs. The personalities of AD's victims are transformed to such an extreme degree that eventually they become strangers to their own families. The changes are devastating. A family will actually lose their loved one to this heart-breaking disorder long before the illness ends the patient's life.

AD gravely impairs a person's ability to carry out any of the ordinary, everyday activities that the rest of us take for granted. Although the mental deterioration is barely detectable at first, eventually the brain becomes so damaged that it can no longer regulate any of the body's systems and eventually death ensues, usually due to infection.

ALZHEIMER'S DISEASE: AN OVERVIEW

Alzheimer's disease is a neurodegenerative disorder that starts silently, invading the brain and triggering a chain of destructive events years before there are noticeable symptoms. Almost imperceptibly it causes memory loss, confusion, poor judgment, language deterioration, and disruptive behavior. The time line of advancement varies from person to person. Early signs of AD, which are forgetfulness and loss of concentration, may be missed because they resemble some of the signs of normal brain aging. AD is the most common form of irreversible dementia and it is always fatal (NIH 2003).

AD is the now is the seventh leading cause of death in the country and the fifth leading cause of death for those over age sixty-five (AA 2007). Although research efforts are more intense than ever before, the cause of the disease is still unknown and there is no cure. It is important to keep in mind though that while there is no cure, there *is* treatment. Furthermore, the sooner a diagnosis is made, the better the chances are that treatment will make an encouraging, if temporary, difference.

AD is a looming public health threat, an equal opportunity catastrophe that currently affects both men and women and spares no racial or ethnic group. Symptoms of AD appear in most people after age sixty-five. However, there are some early-onset forms of the disease seen in 8 percent or less of patients (Smith 2005) that are usually linked to a specific gene defect and that may surface as early as age thirty. Although rare in younger adults, when it does occur in such cases there has generally been a parent or sibling who has also had the illness. The primary risk factor for AD is age, and one out eight individuals sixty-five and older is affected. It is estimated that 50 percent of adults eighty-five and older have AD (NINDS 2004).

Dementia of the Alzheimer's type inflicts unimaginable havoc on affected families, especially for those individuals who are primarily responsible for the care and welfare of the patient. Early on, caregivers feel isolated and hopeless because they are tending to a loved one who has a destructive illness that runs a very dismal course. They also feel lonely because they are cut off from most of the social contacts and leisure activities they once enjoyed. All their time is committed to meeting the basic needs of individuals whose memories and abilities have weakened considerably. Moreover, it soon becomes alarmingly clear that things will only get worse.

From 2000 to 2004, AD deaths increased by 32.8 percent (AA 2007). As the number of individuals with AD swells, so do the legions of overburdened caregivers, those millions of excessively stressed elderly spouses and adult children who shoulder the multiple, oppressive responsibilities that make them so easily susceptible to all manner of emotional, physical, and financial pressure.

More than seven out of ten people with AD live at home and 75 percent of them receive care from family members and friends (NIA 2003). As the disease progresses, families must often use long-term paid care. People with AD live for an average of eight to ten years, and an average lifetime cost per patient is in the high six figures (AA 2007). In 2005 Medicare spent $91 billion on beneficiaries with AD and other dementias. That number is projected to more than double to $189 billion by 2015 (AA 2007).

AD can shorten both total life expectancy and active life expectancy, with different degrees of disability and impairments. Compared with men with AD, female victims spend more years with physical impairments (Dodge and Shen 2003). AD is a major cause of hospitalization among older people and half of all nursing home residents have AD or a related disorder (AA 2007). Some studies have also suggested a strong association between the prevalence of comorbid medical conditions (that is, having simultaneous conditions that are usually independent of each other) and cognitive status among people suffering from AD (Doraiswamy, Leon, and Cummings 2002).

The Alzheimer's Association has recently developed a unique Web tool that helps individuals find the right care options, ranging from home- and community-based care to assisted living and nursing home care. The CareFinder asks for information about a person's needs, abilities, and preferences. After the information is entered, a personalized printout is issued with recommended care options and questions for screening a caregiver or facility. If the patient or caregiver is unsure about a question, he can take the form to a physician or other healthcare provider.

CareFinder provides questions to ask when screening a caregiver or a facility. Go to http://www.alz.org/care finder/index.asp. The CareFinder also provides detailed information on a variety of issues about care options, including planning ahead, resources, and support programs. CareFinder includes Web links to other resources such as the Eldercare Locator, National Academy of Elder Law Attorneys (NAELA), message boards, and chat rooms.

Older men appear to be more likely to experience moderate or severe memory impairment than older women. In 2002, 15 percent of men age sixty-five and over were found to have experienced moderate or severe memory impairment compared to 11 percent of women. At age eighty-five, the difference narrowed and approximately one-third of both men and women experienced moderate or severe memory impairment (EPA 2006).

Memory skills are fundamental to general cognitive functioning, and declining scores on memory tests are indicators of general cognitive loss for older adults. Low cognitive functioning, for example,

Norman, a retired bank official, is a robust sixty-nine-year-old widower whose behavior is worrying his two sons. He has lived alone for several years and always seemed to manage quite well. But for the past several months, the sons have noticed some very troubling signs. Once a well-tailored, fastidious man, Norman now rarely shaves, he wears the same clothes for several days at a time, and is generally unkempt. It's useless to phone him—he is almost unintelligible. When either of his sons offers to help him with personal care or financial matters, he becomes highly agitated and hostile. He calls them "troublemakers" and accuses them of "trying to take over."

With great difficulty the sons finally manage to take Norman to see his primary care physician. After a complete physical and neurological examination, the doctor told the sons that Norman had moderate to severe dementia of the Alzheimer's type. Within three months Norman became incontinent and his unruly behavior escalated. Despite the sons' best efforts to care for their father at home, within six months he was admitted to a nursing home.

memory impairment, is a major risk factor for nursing home placement (Wygaard and Albreksten 1992; Mehta, Yaffe, and Covinsky 2002). Additionally, deficits in activities of daily living, incontinence, and behavioral disturbances are further risk factors for nursing home admission.

The number of Americans with AD will continue to grow. By 2050 the estimates of individuals who will contract the disease range from 11.3 million to 16 million (Hebert et al. 2003). It is also expected that these numbers will soar due to the rapid growth of the elderly population.

Scientists have understood for some time that AD develops as a result of a complex course of events that takes place over a period of time inside the brain and that are influenced by both genetic and non-genetic factors. As the disease evolves, the brain sustains severe damage that distorts memory, thinking, judgment, and behavior. The uncharacteristic behavioral changes can be especially frightening for both the patient and the family. The fear is generated not so much from the prospect of physical pain and suffering but rather from the inescapable loss of all the memories that are the essence of one's identity. Eventually the brain deterioration is so far-reaching that it becomes impossible for the victim to perform everyday activities, or to function independently in the simplest, most basic manner.

At first, a person with AD is terrifyingly aware that something has gone very wrong with his mental abilities. The reactions to this awareness range from paranoia and agitation to denial, hostility, and aggression. Because there is a loss of self-image and initiative, depression commonly coexists with AD. In time the disorder steals not only a person's memory and awareness but also all those distinctive personality traits that characterize and define the individual.

A diagnosis of AD is so alarming for patients and their families that some individuals avoid taking their loved one to the doctor's even when they are convinced something is seriously wrong. They may fear what they will learn, think that nothing can be done, or regard a malfunctioning memory as a normal part of aging. Families have been known to deny there is anything wrong and attribute the behavioral changes to old age, stress, absentmindedness, or "senility."

The far-reaching effects of AD on families have been described as "collateral damage," the military term referring to unintended consequences of battle. This is particularly meaningful to anyone directly involved in fighting AD. While the primary target is the patient, the family also suffers.

"It's a national imperative to find effective means to diagnose, treat and prevent this disease," declared David Banks, RPh, a public health specialist at the FDA's Office of Special Health Issues. "When you look at it demographically, the nearly 80 million baby boomers living in the United States . . . now have an average life expectancy of approximately 78 years. One in five Americans could be age 65 or older by 2030, and tens of millions of baby boomers will live into their 80s. The Alzheimer's Association projects that as many as 14 million Americans could have Alzheimer's disease in 2050. When viewed in the context of accelerating Social Security and Medicare costs . . . , the future monetary costs of Alzheimer's disease may be unsustainable. The human costs could be even greater."

Most of us have only recently become better acquainted with this illness because of the late former president Ronald Reagan's long, well-publicized struggle with AD. An explosion of AD research in the last ten years and the continuing momentum to understand AD contribute to future hopes for potential prevention and treatment strategies. Furthermore, expanded efforts to understand normal brain aging may provide valuable insights for maintaining cognitive function and protecting against dementia.

DISTINGUISHING CHARACTERISTICS OF ALZHEIMER'S DISEASE

The two prominent abnormalities in the brain that characterize Alzheimer's disease are amyloid plaques and neurofibrillary tangles. The plaques, which are found in the tissue between the brain's neurons, are unusual clumps of a protein called beta-amyloid, or a-beta. Decomposing bits of neurons and other cells add to plaque buildup. Neurofibrillary tangles are bundles of twisted strands found inside the neurons. These tangles are largely made up of a protein called tau. In healthy neurons the tau protein contributes to the functioning of microtubules that are essential parts of a neuron's structure and that distribute substances throughout the nerve cell. However, in AD, tau is changed in a way that causes it to twist into pairs of coiled strands that form tangles. When this happens the microtubules cannot work correctly and they collapse. This breakdown of the neuron's transport system damages cell communications and causes them to die (NINDS 2004). Scientists have been debating for decades whether the plaques and tangles are responsible for the degeneration of the neurons in the brain or whether they are just markers indicating where nerve cells have died. For the past several years, the preponderance of evidence indicates both amyloid and tau in causing AD and that amyloid initiates the process of damage and destruction (Wolfe 2006).

DIAGNOSING AND TREATING ALZHEIMER'S DISEASE

It is normal for memory to decline and for the ability to absorb complex information to slow as people grow older. However, AD is not a part of normal aging. A clinician must rule out a number of possible causes of dementia, which can include drug reactions, endocrine disorders, strokes, brain injuries, and depression, in the course of determining a diagnosis. By some estimates, there are roughly one hundred disorders that come under the heading of dementia. But of all the dementias, AD is by far the most common.

Primary care physicians, usually the first healthcare professionals to see elderly patients, have learned to diagnose and treat AD in a timely manner.

- They know how to distinguish dementia from normal age-associated memory impairment.
- Family members are included in the initial doctor's visit. This helps to confirm whether the problems have worsened over time.
- Clinicians screen for loss of function in at least one other cognitive area. This is done because AD patients have problems with language, decision making, planning for the future, or doing calculations. Some typical warning signs are when an individual can no longer balance a checkbook or has trouble remembering recent events, activities, or the names of familiar people or things (Levey 2001).

Today, AD can be diagnosed conclusively only by examining the brain after death. Nevertheless, it is possible to make a strong probable diagnosis on living patients by taking a complete medical history, administering neurological and psychological tests, and doing a physical exam, blood and urine laboratory tests, and a brain-imaging scan.

Once symptoms begin, the disease can be diagnosed with up to 90 percent accuracy by experienced physicians (Bren 2003). Newer research being done based on the analysis of spinal fluid is showing promise in helping confirm the diagnosis (Relkin 2002).

A recently developed imaging test has improved their precision even more. Scientists have learned that testing blood flow in a specific region of the brain combined with clinical assessment may boost the degree of diagnostic certainty in difficult cases to almost 100 percent. The test involves use of single-photon emission computed tomography, SPECT for short (Bonte et al. 2004).

Strategies for Diagnosing AD

- A complete medical history includes information about the person's general health, past medical problems, and any difficulties the person has carrying out daily activities.
- Physical examination helps to rule out treatable causes of dementia and identify signs of other illnesses.
- Medical tests that examine blood, urine, spinal fluid, drug and alcohol use, and thyroid function help doctors find other possible diseases causing the symptoms.
- Neurological tests help identify movement disorders or stroke.
- Neuropsychological tests measure memory, problem solving, attention, counting, and language.
- Imaging studies are also helpful particularly when they are combined with a medical and family history.

TESTING: NEUROPSYCHOLOGICAL AND COGNITIVE TESTS

When evaluating patients suspected of having AD, physicians may use several different tests in order to measure memory, language and math skills, and other competencies related to mental functioning. Everyone understands what is meant by memory and language and math skills, but what is less familiar is another essential competency called *executive functioning*. Most people are easily able to order pizza for delivery. But this simple act would be an insurmountable task for an AD patient. The chances are that the affected individual could not make the call, select the size and topping, then leave his name, address, and telephone number. That is because executive functions, those problem-solving skills and abilities to carry out once-automatic everyday tasks, are seriously damaged.

One of the most common tests clinicians typically use to assess the status of a person with probable dementia is the Mini-Mental State Examination, or MMSE (Folstein, Folstein, and McHugh 1975). The test examines orientation, memory, and attention as well as an individual's ability to name objects, follow verbal and written commands, and copy a complex shape.

Examples of Neuropsychological Tests

Additional tests recommended for the detection of dementia:

- Kokmen Short Test of Mental Status
- Seven-Minute Screen
- Memory Impairment Screen
- Benton Temporal Orientation Test
- Clock-Drawing Test

Source: Petersen 2001

NEUROIMAGING

Changes in the brain's structure and function consistent with AD have been identified through the use of advanced radiology. This type of imaging may also be used to recognize strokes, tumors, or other problems that can cause dementia.

Cortical atrophy, the degeneration of the brain's outer layer, the cortex, is common in many forms of dementia and is usually visible on a brain scan. Normally the appearance of the brain's cortex is very wrinkled with ridges of tissue called *gyri* and deep furrows called *sulci*. In individuals with cortical atrophy the steady progressive loss of neurons causes the ridges to become thinner and the furrows to widen.

As brain cells die, the fluid-filled cavities in the middle of the brain called *ventricles* expand to fill the available space, thus becoming much larger than normal. Brain scans can also identify changes in the brain's structure and function that strongly suggest AD.

Computerized tomographic (CT) scans and magnetic resonance imaging (MRI) are frequently used to help confirm a diagnosis in a patient with suspected dementia. Imaging is also used for other brain disorders such as blood vessel alterations, brain atrophy, stroke, transient ischemic attacks (TIAs, or ministrokes), and subdural hematoma (a traumatic brain injury where blood collects between the outer and middle tissues). There are additional types of scans called *functional brain imaging* that allow researchers to observe the brain as it operates. Although they are seldom used solely as diagnostic tools, such imaging is important in research and ultimately may help to identify people with dementia earlier than is currently possible. In different ways, these scans are able to detect abnormalities of brain function.

Examples of Functional Brain Imaging

- Functional MRI (fMRI)
- Single photon-emission computed tomography (SPECT)
- Positron emission tomography (PET)
- Magnetoencephalography (MEG)

RISK FACTORS FOR ALZHEIMER'S DISEASE

There are two kinds of risk factors for AD: those that can be modified and those over which there is no control, such as age and sex. (Age is the leading known risk factor.) Genetics is a third risk factor that cannot be controlled. Researchers have learned there are genetic links to both early-onset and late-onset AD. Atypical inherited forms of AD can strike as early in individuals who are in their thirties or forties. Mutations on three genes are linked to this rare early-onset form of AD (NIMH 2006). A fourth gene encodes a protein called apolipoprotein E (ApoE) that is linked to late-onset, or sporadic, AD. Almost 25 percent of the population carries a gene called Apoe4, which is linked to an elevated risk of developing late-onset AD (Bertram et al. 2005).

Genetics Home Reference is a guide to understanding genetic conditions, available at http://www.ghr.nlm.nih.gov. This resource provides consumer-friendly information about the effects of genetic variations on human health.

THE "GOLD STANDARD" FOR DIAGNOSING ALZHEIMER'S DISEASE

When the brain of an AD patient is autopsied, the pathologist finds not only brain destruction due to cell death, but also the accumulation neurofibrillary tangles and sticky clumps of plaque that are the hallmarks of the disease. The excessive buildup of the naturally occurring tau protein eventually contributes to the destruction of a once healthy brain. As a result, the patient's ability to function declines. Researchers have found that these formations generally increase in the brain as AD progresses (NINDS 2004).

Drugs Prescribed for Alzheimer's Patients

Tacrine (Cognex, also called THA) was the first drug to be approved. It has been replaced by:

- Donepezil (Aricept)
- Rivastigmine (Exelon)
- Galantamine (Razadyne, previously known as Reminyl).

These three drugs treat mild to moderate AD.

- Memantine (Namenda) blocks glutamate that may hyperstimulate healthy brain cells, causing them to become overactive and die. It is used in combination with cholinesterase inhibitor to treat moderate to severe AD symptoms.

Although there is no cure at this time, there are drugs available to treat the symptoms of AD. Essentially, each of the three FDA-approved drugs acts the same way: they increase the level of acetylcholine, a key chemical in the brain that nerves require in order to communicate successfully with each other.

The drugs target an enzyme called *cholinesterase*, which is responsible for acetylcholine breakdown. By obstructing the enzyme, they are able to protect the integrity of the acetylcholine supply. The cholinesterase inhibitors, the first three drugs listed above often have a positive effect on symptoms because they preserve an adequate supply of acetylcholine that allows better nerve communication. (Also on the list is a fourth FDA-approved drug, Namenda, which is often used in combination with one of the cholinesterase inhibitors.)

Within the last few years, the focus of AD research has shifted from seeking a cure for the disease to concentrating on prevention. Although this is one more advance in the war against AD, it is a limited victory. Current research indicates that although symptoms may improve, the nerve cells are still dying and the scattered, destructive plaques and tangles are still forming. Nonetheless, anyone in the early stages of AD deserves a trial of the medication since there have been many successes that were very rewarding for both patient and caregiver.

Trey Sunderland, MD, chief of the Geriatric Psychiatry Branch of the National Institute of Mental Health (NIMH) notes that people who are on cholinesterase inhibitors tend to go to nursing homes later than people who are not on the drugs (Lopez et al. 2002). In fact, some scientists have reported a delay of as much as twenty-two months in nursing home admission (Provenzano et al. 2001).

In January 2004 the first and only drug approved for treatment of moderate to severe AD became available in the United States. It also was the first time that combination therapy for dementia was recommended (Miller 2004). Memantine, also known by its market name, Namenda, was approved and has been used in Europe for many years to treat people with moderate to severe AD. This drug is thought to act by blocking the action of glutamate, a brain chemical that seems to be overactive in people with AD. Glutamate is the most common neurotransmitter in the brain.

Researchers report potential benefits for patients receiving donepezil plus memantine (Clark and Francis 2005). Dr. Piero G. Antuono, professor of neurology at the Medical College of Wisconsin, explains: "This is extremely important for memory because we know that some typical electric responses of brain cells which are an indication of learning and storing new information are modulated through this chemical called glutamate. What happens in Alzheimer's disease, and possibly also in other degenerative diseases, is that as healthy brain cells die there is an increased release of glutamate which may hyper-stimulate healthy brain cells, causing them to be 'exhausted' or to die." Memantine is used alone or given in combination with one of the cholinesterase inhibitors. The two-pronged approach targets the effects of specific chemicals.

> Namenda was approved by the FDA in October 2003 but it was not available to the public until January 2004.

The argument favoring early diagnosis is all the more persuasive because the medications generally work best early in the course of the disease, and the longer the supportive chemical, acetylcholine, stays in the brain, the longer one's long-term memory stays intact. It is important to understand, however, that only certain patients are successful candidates for these drugs. Many do not respond and others simply cannot tolerate certain side effects.

As a rule, the combination of memantine and one of the aforementioned drugs is the standard treatment doctors use early in the disease in anticipation of significantly improving the patient's quality of life. Memantine is also used in selected moderate to severe AD cases. In any event, researchers have picked up the pace and it appears promising that future scientific investigation will yield more and better treatments that will slow or even stop the progression of AD Although the diagnosis of AD is a bleak one, helpful treatments, widely available support, and promising accelerated research are all encouraging signs for patients and caregivers.

Pharmacological treatments that can prevent or halt the progression of symptoms are still years away. Nonetheless, those who study AD are quick to add that there are measures an individual can take that may help prevent or at least postpone symptoms of the degenerative brain disease by reducing risk factors.

Modification of Potential Risk Factors

- Lowering cholesterol levels
- Lowering high blood pressure levels
- Exercising regularly
- Engaging in intellectually stimulating activities (NIH 2005)

SURVIVAL RATE

After the diagnosis of AD, one of the key questions patients and families ask about is how long the afflicted individual can be expected to live. Unsurprisingly, scientists have learned that people with AD have a significantly decreased survival rate when compared with the average life expectancy of the US population. As an example, men have a median survival of 4.2 years from their initial diagnosis and women have a median survival of 5.7 years (Larson et al. 2004). Men were noted to have poorer survival numbers across all age groups when compared to women.

Other factors, including severity of cognitive impairment, decreased ability to carry out daily activities, history of falls, and chronic illnesses such as diabetes and heart disease, further shortened the life spans of people with AD.

DIAGNOSTIC AND PREVENTION STRATEGIES: BIOLOGICAL MARKERS, HOMOCYSTEINE LEVELS, NEUROIMAGING, AND NEUROPSYCHOLOGICAL TESTS

Alzheimer's research is increasingly focused on the impact of environmental and lifestyle factors. The specific behaviors that scientists have found to be associated with decreasing the chances of developing the disease are lowering cholesterol levels, controlling hypertension, exercising on a regular basis, and engaging in stimulating intellectual activities. Studies of elders engaging in intellectually stimulating activities (such as learning a new language or how to use a computer, playing card games that require strategizing, and solving crossword puzzles), exercising, and consuming wholesome diets are consistent with research about the effects of positive lifestyle behaviors. As an example, there is strong evidence that improvement in brain activity and cognitive function is linked to physical exercise. One such study found that the function of neurons in key parts of the brain increased along with improvements in cardiovascular fitness. The researchers compared a group of physically inactive individuals to a group of walkers and found that the walkers were able to pay better attention and focus more clearly on goals. Scientists offered the possibility that physical activity may be beneficial because it improves blood flow to the brain (Colcombe et al. 2004).

Researchers are also tracking alterations in specific *biological markers* (or *biomarkers*), namely, the levels of biological compounds found in adults in their blood, urine, and cerebrospinal fluid. An example of a biomarker is the tau protein measured in the spinal fluid. This is being done to determine if changes in these markers correspond to early AD changes in the brain. More knowledge of the structure and function of biological markers can improve the focus and effectiveness of drug development that may result in new prevention strategies.

According to research reported in *Stroke: A Journal of Cerebral Circulation*, put out by the American Heart Association, moderate elevations of the biomarker homocysteine, an amino acid, are found to be associated with a greater than fivefold increase in the risk for stroke and almost triple the risk for AD (McIlroy 2002). Homocysteine functions as a building block of protein and normally it is used by the body in cellular metabolism.

The growing population of the elderly is anticipated to cause a rise in the reported incidence of vascular diseases such as atherosclerosis, hypertension, and diabetes. This will lead to an increase in the frequency of vascular dementia. The increase will be highly significant due to the prevalence of AD in these age groups. However, research for the prevention of the dementias is impeded since both Alzheimer's and vascular dementia seem to have several likely causes. Brain deterioration of unknown cause, cardiovascular disorders, and genetic factors have all been implicated.

It has been general knowledge for many years that deficiency of certain vitamins, namely, vitamin B_{12} and folic acid (folate), can cause neurological dysfunction including cognitive impairment. Foods such as fruits, leafy green vegetables, and whole grains are good sources of vitamin B_{12} and folate. In a recent study, higher folate intake was modestly correlated with lower homocysteine levels, indirectly suggesting that a lower homocysteine level is a potential mechanism for the association between higher folate intake and a lower AD risk. But conclusive evidence about the role of increased folate intake and the prevention or slowing down of AD has not yet been demonstrated. Researchers caution that clinical trials must be completed first (Luchsinger et al. 2007).

For a dietary supplement fact sheet on folate, visit http://www.ods.od.nih.gov/factsheets/folate.asp.

Poor diet, which is common not only in old age but also especially among people with dementia, has been associated with high homocysteine levels. And yet, it is also possible that elevated homocysteine levels could be the result of stroke or dementia. However, at this time it is still questionable whether elevated homocysteine levels are the cause or the consequence of stroke and dementia. It is also still unclear whether therapy with any of the B vitamins will reduce the incidence of cerebrovascular disease, AD, or vascular dementia, although researchers acknowledge it is possible (Korczyn 2002).

Certain substances in the blood and cerebrospinal fluid (CSF) may reflect early changes in the brain associated with AD. For example, one biomarker study team found elevated levels of tau and beta-amyloid proteins in the CSF of several research participants who had dementia and a few who had AD. The results of the research were helpful in distinguishing AD from other types of dementia.

Neuroimaging of the brain is another area of investigation that has yielded helpful data. Scientists have been able to note changes in the size of specific areas of the brain that indicate the development of AD (Thompson et al. 2003). The cerebral cortex is the gray matter that covers a large area of the brain. It is the region primarily responsible for memory input into the hippocampus, a tiny organ buried deep in the brain. The hippocampus helps regulate memory and emotion. AD patients sustain marked shrinkage of these areas. It has been determined that the ability to distinguish between normal cognition and mild cognitive impairment is enhanced by using both imaging and biomarker measures combined.

Neuropsychological tests have recently demonstrated their usefulness and value for clinicians. As an example, researchers were interested in learning whether individuals with AD had exhibited signs of cognitive impairment before dementia symptoms began. They studied participants who completed a series of neuropsychological tests over a period of several years, and they learned individuals who were ultimately diagnosed with AD had poorer scores on the initial tests than participants who remained cognitively healthy (Saxton, Lopez, and Ratcliff 2004).

The National Institute of Neurological Disorders and Stroke conducts and supports research on neurodegenerative and dementing disorders, including AD. Current research and study include testing different types of drugs and other substances to determine if AD progression can be halted. Included in the research are nonsteroidal anti-inflammatory drugs (NSAIDS), statins (such as those used for lowering cholesterol), folic acid, and vitamins B_6 and B_{12}. Scientists are also exploring the potential of vaccines. Antioxidants such as vitamin E may protect cells, but the protective influence declines in aging individuals.

Researchers generally agree that finding a treatment that would delay the onset of AD by just five years could reduce the number of those afflicted by nearly 50 percent (Brookmeyer, Gray, and Kawas 1998). The average age for the onset of symptoms is now seventy-five. Dr. Stephen Ferris, executive director of the Aging and Dementia Research Center at New York University, states, "If you can delay symptoms from emerging by only five years, then the average age would be 80 and you would reduce by 50 percent the number of cases." This is because older people would die of other natural causes before they developed AD (Weaver 2004).

Researchers have also expanded the study of normal memory changes due to aging in the hopes of understanding more fully how AD develops. Clearly, an aging brain is a well-known risk factor for AD, and the more that is done to support the health of an older brain, the more researchers can achieve in their investigations of AD. A better understanding of how the brain ages helps scientists develop strategies for maintaining and enhancing cognitive function.

Families and others caring for the AD patient need to know that there are other medications that, while not specific for the disease, can help to control many of the troubling behavioral symptoms of AD such as sleeplessness, agitation, wandering, anxiety, and depression. Treating these symptoms often makes patients more comfortable and that, in turn, makes the quality of life better for both patient and caregiver.

THE GLOBAL MENACE

Dementia is dreaded all over the world because it is a disability that destroys minds, ruins relationships, and eventually kills. The World Health Organization (WHO) estimates that the total number of people worldwide affected by the various forms of dementia has reached more than 29 million. There are currently 18 million people with dementia worldwide, and this number will rise to 34 million in 25 years' time. The increase is due entirely to the rapid aging of populations (Graham 2001).

As life expectancies continue to lengthen and the global population grows, those numbers will double by 2030. Edward Truschke, president of the Alzheimer's Association National Office in the United States, warned that "we have an imminent worldwide epidemic" when referring to the increasing aging population and the prevalence of the disease (Truschke 2000; Ferri et al. 2005).

The situation in the rest of the developed world is similar to that in the United States. AD exacts a huge toll in healthcare costs, disability, and lost productivity of both patients and caregivers. There are powerful social, personal, and financial impacts reflected in global estimates. As an example, the financial burden of dementia, including direct care costs and lost productivity, is projected in the hundreds of billions of dollars annually, an assessment that excludes the cost of direct care by family caregivers. The full effects of AD are truly staggering yet are not well known publicly.

MORE ABOUT THE FINANCIAL ASPECTS OF ALZHEIMER'S DISEASE

Although AD is the most common cause of dementia among people age sixty-five and older, as mentioned earlier, the disease can occur in people in their thirties, forties, or fifties. Although smaller in numbers, individuals who experience early onset have the same symptoms as older adults with the illness. The main difference is the way the disease affects the families of middle-aged adults since so many of them still have parental responsibilities. Consequently, spouses, children, and other close relatives need to understand the behavioral changes they see and how to function together as a family during this time of physical and emotional turmoil.

Patients with early-onset AD are usually still employed. Consequently, there will be issues to face in the workplace since the predictable cognitive decline will certainly affect business relationships and work performance. These younger AD patients typically are viewed as lazy or unstable. As a result they may be terminated for poor performance, willful misconduct, or psychiatric reasons instead of acquiring the diagnosis that could qualify as a medical disability. The subsequent income loss causes a devastating crack in a family's economic base.

However, a much more common, equally disruptive situation occurs when an aging parent has late-onset AD. In such circumstances the primary caregiver is generally a daughter with both family and work obligations in addition to caring for the elderly mother, father, or both. Because of these weighty responsibilities, her work attendance may be poor. She may even have to leave her place of employment temporarily if she is the primary caregiver for aging parents.

American business spends an appalling $61 billion a year on AD, a twofold increase from the amount calculated in 2002 and a dollar amount equivalent to the net profits of the top ten *Fortune* 500 companies. The study, "Alzheimer's Disease: The Costs to US Businesses in 2002," was commissioned by the Alzheimer's Association and released at the Long-Term Care Symposium sponsored by the US Chamber of Commerce. It warns that the cost for US business and the nation will continue to soar as baby boomers hit the highest-risk age for getting the disease.

Study author Dr. Ross Koppel, a researcher and professor at the University of Pennsylvania and president of the Social Research Corporation, provided detailed breakdowns of the $61 billion and calculated that the cost to business of healthcare for people with AD is $24.6 billion, including a business tax contribution to federal healthcare costs and research. The report added that the total cost to businesses of workers who are caregivers for people with AD is $36.5 billion (Koppel 2002). The rough estimates include:

- Absenteeism—$10 billion
- Productivity losses—$18 billion
- Worker replacement cost—$6 billion

- Continuing insurance for workers on leave and temporary worker replacement fees—$2 billion
- Employee Assistance Program usage—$64 million

"We have known for a long time that Alzheimer's disease exacts an enormous economic toll on individuals and families, who exhaust their life savings providing and paying for care, and on state and federal governments that spend billions through Medicare, Medicaid and smaller programs to help pay for health and long-term care," stated Stephen McConnell, former interim president and CEO of the Alzheimer's Association. "Less well known is the financial burden Alzheimer's inflicts on businesses—even though the vast majority of people with the disease are out of the workforce by the time it strikes."

The calculations are based on a pool of 4.5 million people, the number estimated to have had AD in 2002. Within the decade, as baby boomers enter their retirement years, the number with AD will begin to explode to as many as 14 million by the middle of the century. All the resources of families, government, and business combined will not be able to support the financial burden under the current structure.

AD often bankrupts families. The illness's steady progression can last eight to ten years, but many of its victims live twenty years or more after the onset of symptoms. Many of the costs are not covered by Medicare or private insurance (NIH 2003). Medicare pays for one hundred days in a nursing home, assuming that the patient is Medicare eligible. Once Medicare benefits expire the patient has two choices: seek help from the state through the state Medicaid agency or pay out of personal funds.

It is very difficult to qualify for Medicaid payments. Most states have stringent regulations regarding the amount of assets an applicant for Medicaid may have. Typically, such an applicant may not have more than two thousand dollars in assets in order to qualify for Medicaid benefits.

Many people who cannot qualify for Medicare or Medicaid have looked ahead, recognized the potential future problems, and have purchased long-term care insurance to pay for their time in a nursing home. Long-term care policies come in many varieties with a broad array of provisions that may only be applicable to a few people. A thorough evaluation must be made of individual needs at the time of purchase.

THE FUTURE BURDEN

There are nearly 80 million baby boomers in the United States, those individuals born between 1946 and 1964. Considering that their average life expectancy is about seventy-eight years, this means that tens of millions of them may live into their eighties. Based on these statistics, the number of AD patients could range from 11.3 to 16 million by 2050 (Hebert et al. 2003).

With increases in the numbers of patients will come an inevitable increase in costs, some of which are readily apparent. As an example, it is projected that direct costs to Medicare for beneficiaries with AD are expected to increase 75 percent, from $91 billion in 2005 to $160 billion in 2010; Medicaid expenditures on residential dementia care will increase 14 percent from $21 billion in 2005 to $24 billion in 2010 (Lewin Group 2004). However, these figures reveal only the tip of the iceberg. The indirect impact of AD conceals a much larger fiscal toll.

When looked at in the context of accelerating Social Security and Medicare costs, the future monetary burden of AD may be unsustainable. However, the human costs could be even greater. It is impossible to measure the social and emotional effects on a patient's family. Their lives and finances are disrupted by the process of a loved one going through slow degeneration of memory and other intellectual skills while losing the ability to perform the activities of daily living we all take for granted. Families must also deal with bizarre and often unmanageable behavior that generally precipitates nursing home admission. There is indeed a national imperative to find effective means to diagnose, treat, and prevent this disease.

ALZHEIMER'S AND SHARED CHARACTERISTICS
OF OTHER DEMENTIAS

For some time, scientists have realized that a number of devastating diseases such as AD, frontotemporal dementia, and Parkinson's disease are characterized by a collection of proteins, though it differs among the diseases. In AD the proteins are beta-amyloid and tau; in Parkinson's, it is synuclein; and in frontotemporal dementia, it is tau. This would seem to indicate that the pathological processes of these diseases must share some characteristics, although how they overlap is not fully understood. Furthermore, scientists also know that many neurodegenerative diseases share some clinical characteristics. As examples, some AD patients have difficulty moving, which is the most obvious symptom of Parkinson's disease. Many Parkinson's patients also have dementia. Sleep-wake disorders, delusions, psychiatric disturbances, and memory loss occur in all of these diseases.

In conclusion, what is clear is that all of these diseases develop over many years and they occur as a result of complex interactions of genes, lifestyle practices, environmental factors, and dynamic features that affect all parts of the body.

Chapter 4

Depression

More Than Just the Blues

*F*ostering an understanding of healthy aging is essential to better care and better well-being for older Americans. All too often, for example, older individuals and their doctors accept depression as a normal part of aging when it is not (Lebowitz et al. 1997). This belief is especially unfortunate for those who develop depression for the first time late in life, when such passivity can prevent the individual from receiving effective care (HHS 2003).

Of the nearly 35 million Americans age sixty-five years and older, an estimated 2 million have a depressive illness and another 5 million may have depressive symptoms that fall short of meeting full diagnostic criteria for a disorder (Conwell 2001).

About 15 percent of older Americans are depressed, and among elders with a chronic illness such as cancer, AD, stroke, or arthritis, the figure increases by another 10 percent (AAGP 2001). However, in spite of such ominous figures, depression continues to be underdiagnosed and undertreated in the community.

Everybody feels sad from time to time, and when the sad feelings pass people move on with their lives. However, persistent sadness is not normal at any age. Living in a state of unremitting melancholy is never a usual feature of the aging process. It may, however, be a sign of clinical depression, and if that is the case, there are treatments available that can make a major improvement in one's well-being and quality of life. To ignore this is to ignore a significant health threat.

The National Institute of Mental Health has targeted both depression and AD for aggressive, expanded research. An estimated 6 percent of people ages sixty-five and older in a given year, or approximately 2 million individuals in this age group, have a diagnosable depressive illness. Furthermore, the evidence suggests that about 40 percent of older adults with major depression also meet the criteria for anxiety, an emotional disorder that is strongly related to several chronic illnesses such as cardiovascular, pulmonary, and endocrine disorders, cancer, AD, and Parkinson's disease (AAGP 2004).

> Depression can be a side effect of certain medications. Older adults are at increased risk for drug reactions because they take more drugs than younger individuals. Seniors buy 30 percent of all prescription drugs and 40 percent of all over-the-counter drugs (FDA 2003).

Depression is one of the most common psychiatric disorders among the elderly. According to a recent study, the highest rates of the disorder were found in long-term care settings, where 30 to 50 percent of the elderly residents were afflicted (Merck 2000). Earlier information revealed that major depression strikes 20 percent of all AD patients, 27 percent of stroke victims, and 11 percent of patients with general dementias (Neel 1996). Clearly, researchers have known for a long time that the disorder is a widespread geriatric health issue.

Statistics from NIMH also show that more than 50 percent of the time, physicians miss or misdiagnose depression in older adults (Ross 2000). Diagnosing depression in the elderly is a challenge because the illness is subtle and the customary symptom, sadness, may be missing.

More commonly, a depressed senior may display a few of the early behaviors associated with dementia such as difficulty paying attention, apathy, and inability to concentrate. Irritability, fatigue, sleep disturbances, and loss of interest in hobbies, particularly in elderly men, are other diagnostic clues.

Older adults are particularly sensitive to stigma about mental illness. When a patient with late-life depression sees a clinician, typically he will describe a variety of physical complaints, for example, headaches, fatigue, gastrointestinal issues, and vague pain. Such symptoms correlate accurately with the signs of a variety of chronic illnesses commonly found in older adults and may seem more tolerable to the elderly patient. Paradoxically, many of those most in need of the physician's help will downplay their symptoms and simulate a cheerful mood while concealing their difficulties.

It is well known that most older adults are living with chronic illnesses as well as a variety of social and economic issues. Consequently, families and many healthcare professionals sometimes mistakenly conclude that depression is the normal result of these problems—an attitude that is often shared by patients themselves. Taken together, these factors have contributed a great deal to the underdiagnosis and undertreatment of depressive disorders in older adults. Depression can and should be treated when it coexists with other illnesses because untreated depression may not only delay recovery from these illnesses but it also can influence their outcome.

Regrettably, late-life depression is often unnoticed and when left untreated the cost in terms of pain, disability, and death is alarmingly high. Moreover, even though effective treatment exists, there are still barriers to identifying and treating this disorder as well as some of the other mental and emotional illnesses in older adults.

Among adults over sixty, depression is one of the eight most disabling medical conditions, *including* heart disease. The most recent data available estimate that depression costs the United States between $30 and $44 billion annually in lost productivity, medical expenses, and premature death (Stewart et al. 2003).

By some estimates, as many as one-sixth of elderly Americans suffer from clinical depression. Moreover, elderly individuals are more likely than younger ones to be troubled by the perceived shame of depression and emphasize physical symptoms instead of psychological ones to their primary care physicians (PCPs). They are also more apt to limit their treatment to their PCPs. The fact that the prescribing of antidepressants has more than doubled between 1985 and 1999 attests to this (Harman et al. 2003).

The effects of late-life depression on older adults are especially destructive for the following reasons:

- It is the most reliable predictor of suicide in the elderly. Although they represent only 13 percent of the US population, individuals age sixty-five and older accounted for 18 percent of all suicide deaths in 2000 (OSP 2005).
- It is a highly significant cause of disability and poor quality of life.
- When it coexists with physical disorders, the prognosis is poor.
- The illness increases the use of healthcare providers and facilities, which contributes to escalating healthcare costs.

DEPRESSION: UNDERDIAGNOSED AND UNDERTREATED

Despite the high prevalence of depressive symptoms and major depressive episodes, late-life depression continues to be overlooked by many healthcare providers. One of the reasons this occurs is because clinicians often wrongly presume that because elders have so many physical illnesses and social and economic problems, depression is a normal consequence of the aging process (NIH 1991). Also, older adults are more likely than most people to want to "handle matters themselves."

Elderly individuals typically have multiple coexisting medical conditions that can delay or obscure the diagnosing of depression. As listed in the current American Psychiatric Association's *Diagnostic and Statistical Manual* (DSM-III-R), some key criteria for the diagnosis of depression include: (1) changes in appetitive or weight, (2) disturbed sleep, (3) fatigue or loss of energy, (4) lack of interest in usual activities, (5) difficulty with concentration, (6) feelings of worthlessness, and (7) suicidal thinking or attempts. Although a minimum of five symptoms are required in order to qualify for a diagnosis of major depression, several of the symptoms are also indicative of a number of common chronic illnesses.

There are multiple other reasons why depression in the elderly is often missed or simply ignored. As mentioned earlier, the signs of late-life depression characteristically consist of irritability, confusion, or inattention. Such behavior seems to be an atypical display of the disorder and consequently the diagnosis is more difficult to make because clinicians, patients, and families frequently credit these symptoms simply to old age. Another suggestion from researchers is that we do not fully understand the degree of intensity of the illness because so many of us have low expectations of seniors in their post-retirement years. We are inclined to underestimate their ability to contribute to society and we frequently undervalue their wisdom and experience. Past research has shown that many elders themselves share this view (Coupland et al. 1988).

Once identified, depression can usually be treated successfully, either with medication, psychotherapy, or a combination of both. When a diagnosis is reached, 80 percent of clinically depressed individuals, including older adults, can be effectively treated by medication, psychotherapy, electroconvulsive therapy (ECT), or a combination of the three. Medication is effective for a majority of people with depression. There are four groups of antidepressants that have been used to effectively treat depressive illness: tricyclics, monoamine oxidase inhibitors (MAOIs), selective serotonin reuptake inhibitors (SSRIs), and norepinephrine and serotonin reuptake inhibitors (NSRIs). Medication compliance is particularly important, but it can be a problem among older patients. It has been estimated that approximately 70 percent of these patients fail to take 25 to 50 percent of their medication (Jeste 2003). Naturally, not all patients respond to the same therapy, and virtually all treatments have side effects. The choice of treatment may depend on the types of side effects that can be best tolerated by that individual.

Depression in the older adult has the potential to disrupt family life as well as threaten the life of the patient. Sadly, most of this suffering is unnecessary because it is widely known that treatment can be effective. Why, then, are there so many untreated elderly individuals? The reasons are wide-ranging:

- Symptoms are easily misinterpreted by clinicians since they are usually described as physical complaints.
- Specific symptoms are treated rather than their underlying cause.
- The symptoms are often so disabling that the distressed individuals cannot accurately describe their emotional pain and ask for help.
- Patients are reluctant to admit to a mental illness because of the perceived stigma and they may delay timely treatment or even refuse help outright.

Not only does depression often exist simultaneously with other illnesses but there are also medications that can trigger its onset. Two classifications of drugs that are used extensively in the elderly population and can produce such an effect are antihypertensives and H_2 blockers (prescribed for stomach acid control). Both have been implicated at one time or another as causes of depression. Mood changes and gloominess have also been linked to corticosteroids, steroid-based anti-inflammatory drugs elders may take for arthritis (MacNair 2006). What's more, the seeds of depression are frequently sown as an aging individual becomes impaired with the onset of certain sensory weaknesses, chiefly, advancing vision and hearing deficits, and all that they imply.

Older adults, just like everybody else, experience the periods of sadness well known to all of us as the "blues." However, these mood changes are usually temporary and benign. As time passes and with the support of family and friends, the discomforting emotions are less distressing. Rarely is further intervention needed or even anticipated.

Ernie is a seventy-five-year-old grandfather with moderate hearing loss. He acquired hearing aids a year ago, but often neglects to wear them. Instead, most of the time he relies on other ways to conceal his impairment. He thought he was managing rather well until the last time he went to his daughter's home to pick up his four-year-old grandson as was his custom each Thursday. As soon as he stepped into her house, his daughter told him that she was reluctantly canceling the weekly trips to the park. "I'm sorry, Dad, I just don't think it's safe to let you take Tyler. You might not hear him call if he needs you." Ernie was stunned. Two years ago he lost his wife of fifty-one years, and the relationship with his grandson was a treasured source of comfort and joy. When he and the boy were together, he reveled in the child's happiness and enjoyed a respite from his grief.

Since the special tie between him and his grandson was so abruptly transformed, Ernie has been overcome with feelings of guilt and worthlessness. He is withdrawn, apathetic, and dwells on feeling that in some way he is being punished. His family, although troubled by his lethargy and increasing confusion, attributes the changes in his behavior to old age.

However, clinical depression is much more serious and prolonged. Families, friends, and healthcare providers need to understand that this situation is not simply a personal weakness that could be changed if the individual would only make an effort. The stricken person is genuinely ill and consequently it is pointless to urge him to "pull himself together" or to suggest that he could "try harder" to recover from a long-lasting sorrow. Such advice might be compared to suggesting that a cancer patient ought to try controlling tumor growth with willpower.

CAUSES OF LATE-LIFE DEPRESSION

When depression occurs in late life, it may be a relapse of an earlier depression. However, if it is a first-time occurrence, the chances are it could have been triggered by another illness, hospitalization, or nursing home placement. Unlike the onset of depression in younger persons, depression in the elderly is thought to be a psychological disorder generated by specific stressors, such as medical illness, physical impairment, or grief following the death of a loved one (Kurlowicz 2003).

There is no one specific cause of depression. For some, a single event can induce the illness while a number of people will develop depressive symptoms for no readily apparent reason. This disease often strikes individuals who felt fine for years until they suddenly had to struggle with a death in the family or a serious illness. Unrelieved stress can take an emotional as well as physical toll in the form of anxiety, depression, or high blood pressure and heart disease. If unattended, stress can seriously damage physical health, psychological well-being, and relationships with friends, family, and coworkers (Smith 1991).

In other situations differences in brain chemistry can affect an individual's mood and cause feelings of despair. Very often individuals who are living in unrelieved, stressful situations (caregivers are a typical and increasingly familiar example) can fall prey to depression.

It is easy to understand why people with serious illnesses, such as cancer, diabetes, heart disease, or stroke, become depressed. They worry constantly about how their illness will change their lives and affect their families. Furthermore, fatigue and discomfort also make it difficult to deal with the symptoms. Genetics, too, can play a role because emerging research has shown that depression is seen in families (Zubenko 2001). If this is the case, the children of depressed parents may be at an increased risk for the illness.

As more research reveals, depression is a serious and often dangerous medical condition, and older adults seem to be especially vulnerable. Regrettably for this population, the vague, obscure symptoms are serious diagnostic obstacles.

Barriers to Timely Diagnosis

- Depressed moods are less noticeable in older adults.
- Some of the symptoms, for example, sleeplessness and poor appetite, also occur in people who are not depressed.
- Physicians who are not psychiatrists may not be adequately trained to diagnose depressive illness.
- Depressed elders usually describe their complaints in terms of bodily ailments.

Symptoms such as social withdrawal, confusion, reduced energy, sleep disturbances, alterations in appetite, and memory impairment apply to both dementia and depression. Furthermore, dementia and depression often coexist. However, it is also very important to understand that a dementia caused by depression is highly likely to be *reversible*. When the depression is treated, confusion and memory problems often clear up. Even if the physician determines that the patient has both depression and an *irreversible* dementia, the depression should be treated.

Depression Link to Dementia

Many patients with dementia triggered by depression show improvement when depression is treated (Jankowiak 2002).

Families and friends concerned about an older adult who is close to them need to reject the myth of senility and be alert for signs of depression. It is always in the patient's best interest to arrange for a thorough medical assessment when the symptoms persist. Delaying or ignoring the evidence can result in intensified physical problems, disability, needless suffering, and ultimately, premature death.

SIGNS OF DEPRESSION

Depression can soon overwhelm a person if no one recognizes the warning signs and takes action. This is especially true in the case of older adults who generally are managing at least one chronic illness, have noticeably diminished strength and vigor, no longer have full-time, productive careers, and have lost several cherished friends and family members over the years. Initially, these normal lifetime experiences will cause sadness.

Nevertheless, after going through a period of grief and feeling distressed, most elders do get back to their daily lives with emotionally healthy attitudes, whereas untreated individuals with clinical depression may not improve for months, years, or at all.

> Because the symptoms of late-onset or geriatric depression are so distinctive, researchers have established that combined treatment approaches, using state-of-the-art pharmacologic and psychotherapeutic techniques, are the preferred management strategies (Pies and Rogers 2005).

Figure 4.1. Common Warning Signs of Depression

- Continuous sadness, anxiety, a hollow feeling
- Fatigue, inactivity, apathy
- Disinterest in daily activities; loss of pleasure in formerly enjoyable activities, including sex
- Changes in sleep patterns; sleeping too much or having trouble getting to sleep
- Eating too much or lack of appetite
- Frequent or excessive crying
- Unrelieved aches and pains after medical treatment; irritability
- Difficulty making decisions; inability to focus; memory problems
- Feelings of hopelessness and guilt
- Thoughts of death; suicide attempt or talking about an attempt

If there is no improvement in the warning signs after a few weeks, the individual should be evaluated by a clinician.

Families and caregivers need to pay particular attention to the subtle indications that their loved one may need prompt medical intervention because occasional changes for the better can be misleading. A depressed individual, for example, may smile and seem friendly while talking to a clinician or when a family member visits, but what seems to be an improvement is temporary. The warning signs must be taken seriously because at best, untreated clinical depression will exacerbate any health problems the person has and at worst it can lead to suicide. Research has shown that more than 90 percent of people who kill themselves have depression or another diagnosable mental or substance abuse disorder (Conwell and Brent 1995; Moscicki 2001).

Suicide is a major public health problem that is preventable. It is one of the top ten leading causes of death in the United States, ranking eighth or ninth since the mid-1990s (SG 1999). Older adults are disproportionately likely to die by suicide. Although they composed only 13 percent of the US population, individuals age sixty-five and older accounted for 18 percent of all suicides in 2000. Among the highest rates (when categorized by gender and race) are white men age eighty-five and older: they account for 59 deaths per 100,000 persons, more than five times the national US rate of 10.6 per 100,000 (OSP, NCIPC, and CDC 2000; Miniño et al. 2002).

The tragedy is that many who went on to commit suicide *did* reach out for help. Studies have shown that about 70 percent of elderly suicide victims had seen a primary care physician in the last month of life, and about 40 percent had seen one in the week prior to taking their own life (NIMH 2003).

GETTING THE NEEDED HELP

Many people are uncomfortable discussing the sensitive subject of mental disorders and consequently are reluctant to admit that someone in their family needs help for an emotional problem. Older adults in particular may view such illnesses as signs of weakness or even taboo—something that is simply not talked about. Families and friends may think they are being helpful when they urge the depressed individual to "snap out of it" or to "be thankful for what you have." Neither statement is supportive, much less helpful.

The first step toward getting help is to acknowledge there is a problem and make an appointment with a primary care physician. After a comprehensive physical examination to rule out other illnesses or possible drug reactions, the doctor may suggest a meeting with a mental health specialist such as a counselor, psychologist, or psychiatrist.

As with most health issues there are often financial concerns involved. However, therapy is generally covered by insurance. Another alternative is to use community health agencies that arrange for treatment at no cost in some situations or with fees based on a sliding scale.

WHEN BEREAVEMENT BECOMES DEPRESSION

Loss of a spouse is common in late life and bereavement is a natural response to the death of a loved one. Universally recognizable features are crying, sorrow, anxiety, agitation, insomnia, and loss of appetite. Research indicates that at some point during the first year of bereavement, about one-fifth of all widows and widowers will experience a major depression, while nearly a third will experience depression for the *entire* first year. Furthermore, all bereaved individuals are susceptible to a range of anxiety disorders and depressive symptoms. The effects of a loss, therefore, present scores of important challenges for treatment (SG 1999).

Clinicians have long known from studies of widowed older adults that this group experiences a higher rate of healthcare use. Causes include an upsurge in hip fractures, more nutritional deficiencies, and increases in functional impairments (Browne, O'Doherty, and McGee 1997; Levine 1997; Peterson 2000). The bereaved often have difficulty handling finances, managing medications, and performing household tasks. Some may even neglect daily routines such as bathing, dressing, and eating. Although the surviving spouse will usually focus on physical ailments, for example, headache, fatigue, and vague complaints of pain, that individual is still increasingly vulnerable to emotional and psychological disorders. Naturally, all physical symptoms need to be explored since any one of them might suggest a health problem that requires further scrutiny. In addition, it is also appropriate to assess cognitive function at this time because researchers have noted that in many cases, it is only *after* a spouse dies that the full extent of a deficit or impairment becomes clear (Mor, McHorney, and Sherwood 1986; Husaini 1997; Prigerson et al. 1997; Chen et al. 1999).

After sustaining the loss of a loved one, bereaved individuals can strengthen their mental and emotional health by cultivating or renewing relationships with family and friends. As a matter of fact, grief counselors and other therapists recommend developing new social connections. Yet this can be very hard to do, particularly if an older adult has any vision or hearing difficulties, mobility problems, or some indication of a cognitive impairment. Besides, these may not be the only problems a bereaved individual faces. There often are more worrisome issues to contend with that frequently surface after a death, such as reduced income, disturbing changes within the family structure, or the threat of an involuntary move, perhaps to an assisted living community or a nursing home.

Bereavement is not a mental health disorder, but if not attended to, it has serious mental health and other health consequences. So what is the best way for family and friends to help in these situations? Initially, the greatest need is that of reassurance, preferably by someone who is able to convey the comforting feelings of full support and genuine concern. The days and weeks following the death of a spouse are filled with constant disruptions and stressful decisions. These range from organizing a funeral to dealing with financial matters and the impact of the loss on family and friends. It is particularly important that someone listen to the bereaved talk about their loss and to accept mourning without criticism. On a practical level, an elderly individual may also need extra help with household tasks, managing finances, and coping with the voluminous paperwork that a death generates.

Helpful bereavement links:

http://www.funerals.org/faq/grieving.htm
http://www.aarp.org/family/lifeafterloss

SUBSTANCE ABUSE AND DEPRESSION

A substantial and growing percentage of older adults misuse alcohol, prescription drugs, or other substances. The number of older adults in need of substance abuse treatment is estimated to more than double from 1.7 million in 2000 and 2001 to 4.4 million in 2020 (Bartels et al. 2005).

Many of the medical and psychiatric disorders that lead to increasing rates of healthcare use by older people are driven by alcohol consumption. These conditions include harmful medication interactions, injury, depression, memory problems, liver disease, cardiovascular disease, cognitive changes, and sleep problems (Liberto, Oslin, and Ruskin 1992; Gambert and Katsoyannis 1995).

Alcoholism and drug abuse can also cause depression. According to a report from the Center for Substance Abuse Treatment/Mental Health Services Administration (http://www.samhsa.gov), the misuse and abuse of legal drugs affects 17 percent of adults age sixty and older. The report goes on to say that since a third of the seniors who abuse alcohol did not have an alcohol abuse problem when they were younger, the implication is that conditions or situations encountered during the aging process were probably in some way responsible for the destructive behavior.

Elderly alcoholics seem to be a "hidden" population who are

easily overlooked by health professionals. The disorder is seldom recognized in older adults and consequently it is less likely to be treated. Another contributing factor is that older drinkers are more socially isolated than younger drinkers. This further obscures the detection of alcoholism because it make the signs of alcohol abuse much harder to recognize. At the same time, there is the tendency of many healthcare providers and families of older adults to mistakenly view some of the signs of alcohol abuse, such as apathy, confusion, and social withdrawal, as more stereotypical signs of aging.

Elders are also more liable to mix drugs and alcohol and consequently they are at high risk for the harmful effects of these combinations. Studies report that older persons regularly consume on average between two and six prescription medications and between one and three over-the-counter medications (Larsen and Martin 1999). Individuals sixty-five and older make up less than 15 percent of the population yet they consume nearly a third of the nation's prescription drugs (Reed 2007).

Antibiotics and drugs for hypertension and heart disease are their most common prescriptions, but they are also taking countless medicines for pain, incontinence, and digestive disorders. Further emphasizing the gravity of the situation is the evidence that, according to at least one pharmacological analysis, antidepressant use among the geriatric population doubled between 1985 and 1999 (Harman, Crystal, and Walkup 2003).

Older adults are also more highly susceptible to the side effects of drugs than younger adults, and adverse events are known to escalate in severity with advancing age. Late-onset alcohol problems also occur in some retirement communities, where drinking at social gatherings is often the norm (Atkinson, Tolson, and Turner 1990) and an unexpected 49 percent of those in nursing homes meet the criteria for alcohol abuse (Joseph 1997). Combined difficulties with alcohol and medication misuse may affect nearly 20 percent of older Americans (Bucholz et al. 1995; NIAAA 1998).

The interactions between alcohol and medications are of particular easily overlooked by health professionals. The disorder is seldom recognized in older adults and consequently it is less likely to be treated. Another contributing factor is that older drinkers are more socially isolated than younger drinkers. This further obscures the detection of alcoholism because it make the signs of alcohol abuse much harder to recognize. At the same time, there is the tendency of many healthcare providers and families of older adults to mistakenly view some of the signs of alcohol abuse, such as apathy, confusion, and social withdrawal, as more stereotypical signs of aging.

Elders are also more liable to mix drugs and alcohol and consequently they are at high risk for the harmful effects of these combinations. Studies report that older persons regularly consume on average between two and six prescription medications and between one and three over-the-counter medications (Larsen and Martin 1999). Individuals sixty-five and older make up less than 15 percent of the population yet they consume nearly a third of the nation's prescription drugs (Reed 2007).

Antibiotics and drugs for hypertension and heart disease are their most common prescriptions, but they are also taking countless medicines for pain, incontinence, and digestive disorders. Further emphasizing the gravity of the situation is the evidence that, according to at least one pharmacological analysis, antidepressant use among the geriatric population doubled between 1985 and 1999 (Harman, Crystal, and Walkup 2003).

Older adults are also more highly susceptible to the side effects of drugs than younger adults, and adverse events are known to escalate in severity with advancing age. Late-onset alcohol problems also occur in some retirement communities, where drinking at social gatherings is often the norm (Atkinson, Tolson, and Turner 1990) and an unexpected 49 percent of those in nursing homes meet the criteria for alcohol abuse (Joseph 1997). Combined difficulties with alcohol and medication misuse may affect nearly 20 percent of older Americans (Bucholz et al. 1995; NIAAA 1998).

The interactions between alcohol and medications are of particular toms are not the ones typically seen in younger adults. Furthermore, there is always the risk of clinicians and families attributing the signs of alcohol abuse to the aging process. This problem of underidentification is further compounded by family members and professional providers who share the misperception that impaired judgment and apathy is a normal part of aging (Gallo, Ryan, and Ford 1999).

The costs of alcoholism and its effects on older adults and their families have the potential to create an enormous financial burden for the Medicare program. The numbers of alcoholic elderly are expected to increase due to the hordes of baby boomers entering old age and, moreover, because this particular generation also has higher rates of substance abuse than any previous generation. For more information visit the Web site of the National Institute of Alcohol Abuse and Alcoholism at http://www.niaaa.nih.gov.

WHEN HELP IS REFUSED

Ordinarily, an alcoholic cannot be forced to get help. However, there are exceptions, such as the occurrence of a violent incident that results in court-ordered treatment or the event of a medical emergency.

Instead of waiting for a loved one to "hit rock bottom," many alcoholism treatment specialists suggest specific practical measures that can lead to treatment. As a first step, families are urged to stop making excuses and to immediately cease protecting the alcoholic, thereby ensuring that the individual experiences the full consequences of drinking to excess. Primary care physicians and clergy members are usually successful at directing older problem drinkers to appropriate social service agencies. It is worth noting that older alcoholic adults have more success with treatment than any other age group; once they decide to seek help, they generally stay with the treatment program.

For more information call the National Drug and Alcohol Treatment Referral Routing Service (Center for Substance Abuse Treatment) at 1-800-662-HELP, or write to:

National Institute on Alcohol Abuse and Alcoholism (NIAAA)
5635 Fishers Lane MSC 9304
Bethesda, MD 20892-9304

Also available online at http://www.niaaa.nih.gov

TREATMENT OPTIONS

Depression can be successfully treated by both mental health specialists and primary care physicians. Allowing that different people require different therapies, there are several options available to clinicians. Antidepressants, for example, can improve mood, enhance concentration, and relieve sleep disturbances. Nevertheless, caregivers must be mindful of the fact that giving medication to elderly patients for depression treatment will remain an ongoing challenge for several reasons:

- Older adults take much longer to achieve a noticeable improvement.
- Drug dosage needs to be very carefully calculated so that it will be therapeutic and not toxic.
- Many elders are noncompliant with a drug regimen and the National Institute of Mental Health estimates that about 70 percent of elderly patients do not take 25 to 50 percent of their medication. A responsible person needs to ensure that the prescription is taken as ordered.

There are additional depression treatment choices available for older adults. Talk therapies are useful and they often are particularly beneficial when used concurrently with drug treatment. Support groups, both formal (those using a trained facilitator) and informal (with family and friends), can supply both new coping skills and many social benefits.

Clinicians also have therapeutic psychosocial strategies to offer, and these approaches can be very effective when treating depression. Research has shown that certain types of short-term psychotherapy, particularly *cognitive-behavioral therapy* (CBT) and *interpersonal therapy* (IT), are effective treatments for late-life depression (Lebowitz, Pearson, and Schneider 1997). Cognitive-behavioral therapy tries to help a person identify then change the negative thinking patterns that contribute to depression. Interpersonal therapy focuses on effective interactions with other people in order to improve relationships. The goal of both therapies is to reduce depressive symptoms. Furthermore, psychotherapy alone has been shown to prolong periods of good mental and physical health. In one study approximately 80 percent of older adults with depression recovered with a combination of treatments (Little et al. 1998). This was also found to be more effective in reducing recurrences of depression (Reynolds et al. 1999).

These interventions may be used either alone or in combination with antidepressant medication. The evidence is clear that with proper treatment, elders can benefit from diminished recurrence of symptoms and enjoy substantial improvement in their emotional state and quality of life (Rupke, Blecke, and Renfrow 2006).

In addition to drug and talk therapies, another treatment used in managing the depression of older adults is electroconvulsive therapy (ECT). This treatment is commonly used in depressed elderly because the response rates for antidepressant drugs in elders are lower than in younger adults. There is, however, a significant drawback to using ECT in the elderly—the potential for seizures. Both risks and benefits need to be weighed by a physician.

Both ECT and antidepressant treatment need to be studied carefully by patients and caregivers because of the risk factors such as confusion, cognitive deficits, and coexisting medical problems. For a full, illustrated explanation of electroconvulsive therapy, see www .medlineplus.gov. The National Institute of Mental Health (NIMH) is another valuable resource for information about these treatments.

Understand that individuals will vary in their responses to treatments for depression. If the symptoms have not improved after several weeks, then the patient should be reassessed and the treatment plan revised.

MORE ABOUT SYMPTOMS

One in five Americans will have a mental illness during their lifetime that is severe enough to require treatment, and many more have problems that prevent them from enjoying their lives. Asking for help is not an easy thing to do, and individuals who are looking for help, either for themselves or a loved one, may become intimidated when they finally visit their healthcare provider.

In order to help people form meaningful questions about their mood and behavioral concerns and to encourage useful discussions between patients and clinicians, log on to the National Institute of Mental Health's Web site at www.nimh.nih.gov. The institute recommends that the following symptoms be looked into by a healthcare professional:

Figure 4.2. Significant Symptoms of Depression

Emotional Symptoms	Physical Symptoms
Anxiety	Sleeping more or less than usual
Feelings of guilt	Eating more or less than usual
Obvious lack of interest in formerly enjoyable experiences	Recurring headaches, stomachaches
Restlessness, irritability	Excessive fatigue
Feelings of worthlessness, of being unloved	Chronic pain
Feelings of despair	Lethargy, indifference

Research has shown that there is a variety of patterns of clinical and biological features among older adults with depression (Lebowitz, Pearson, and Schneider 1997). When compared with elderly individuals whose depression began in early adulthood, those whose first depressive episode appears in late life are likely to have a more chronic course of illness. Furthermore, there is growing evidence that depression beginning in late life is associated with vascular changes in the brain (NIMH 2003).

TREATMENT WITH MEDICATION

Both antidepressants and short-term psychotherapies have been found to be effective treatment options for late-life depression (Lebowitz 1997). Existing antidepressants are known to influence the functioning of certain neurotransmitters in the brain. The newer medications, chiefly the selective serotonin reuptake inhibitors (SSRIs), are generally preferred over the older medications, including tricyclic antidepressants (TCAs) and monoamine oxidase inhibitors (MAOIs), because they have fewer and less severe side effects (Reynolds et al. 1999). Both generations of medications are effective in relieving depression, although some individuals respond better to one than the other.

> About one in five elderly patients receive a prescription for a drug that is *inappropriate* for them to use. Two antidepressants, amitriptyline and doxepin, top the list of inappropriate medications, according to a study reported in the August 2005 issue of the *Archives of Internal Medicine* (James 2005).

Other factors that contribute to the development of the disorder are:

- Antidepressants may take several weeks to effect a noticeable change. Once the depression improves, clinicians may advise continuing the medication for a period of time. All too often older adults simply get additional drugs without a reassessment of their previous prescriptions, a practice that can be hazardous. In order to guard against potential drug reactions, all consumers need to act responsibly and inform their physicians about their medications before accepting any new drug prescriptions. This means any over-the-counter products, including all vitamins and herbal supplements.
- Individuals on an antidepressant regimen must take these drugs exactly as prescribed, and this requires a firm commitment by both patient and family members. Since any real progress may not be noticed for several weeks and some drugs have unwelcome side effects (most commonly dry mouth, constipation, and occasionally weight gain), continued support and encouragement is essential in order to help the individual stay with the treatment plan.

Many side effects can be managed successfully without more drugs. For example, constipation and weight gain can be controlled by paying careful attention to diet and fluid intake and by exercising regularly. An additional benefit of exercise is that it boosts serotonin levels, which in turn promotes a feeling of well-being. Another annoying side effect, dry mouth, can be relieved by using sugarless gum or sugar-free hard candies and by drinking more water.

Caution: The use of herbs as a treatment alternative has kindled much active interest by both consumers and professionals. In Europe, St. John's Wort (*Hypericum perforatum*) has been widely used for many years to treat depression. Yet it has not gained the same degree of acceptance in the United States. Furthermore, in 2000 the FDA issued a public health advisory warning that the herb appears to affect a key metabolic pathway used by many drugs used to treat such conditions as heart disease, depression, certain cancers, and transplant rejection. Patients should *not* take herbal supplements without consulting a physician. The National Center for Complementary and Alternative Medicine and the Food and Drug Administration have joined forces to conduct studies of this herbal remedy.

DEPRESSION AND THE BURGEONING SENIOR POPULATION

Depression may be even more common among baby boomers than those born before World War II. Recent evidence suggests that risks for depression are also higher for women, and for separated or divorced people (Hasin, Weissman, Mazure 2005). Regrettably, fewer than a third of those with clinical depression actually try to get help even though there is a broad range of proven treatments available.

The National Institute of Mental Health and related agencies are committed to promoting public health policies that educate people that treating depression does work. What's more, specialists in the field point to the fact that there are even new research findings suggesting the possibility of preventing the disease by identifying people very early in the course of depression and screening others who are at risk.

As depression is generally accompanied by dependency and disability, it causes great distress for the affected individual and his family. Although the research indicates that while most afflicted elders have been suffering from episodes of the illness during much of their lives, for others, a late-life onset is the first indication of the disorder. Significantly, this even includes individuals in their eighties and nineties (AAGP 2004).

Since the outcome of depression therapy is largely positive, it is hard to understand why so many depressed older adults are not treated. Scientific investigation has yielded many studies that clearly show depression to be brain disorder, and there is every indication that when treatment is effective, the brain actually changes. Nevertheless, despite all the evidence, there are still too many people who view depression as a normal part of growing old. It is encouraging to note that intensive efforts by healthcare professionals are slowly changing this false perception of the illness.

WHY DEPRESSION IS OFTEN UNTREATED

At one time researchers thought that depression was solely a chemical imbalance caused by an inadequate supply of certain neurotransmitters, the chemicals used to send messages throughout the cell network of the brain. But new information has changed that view. It is now known that the relationship between depression and the way our minds and bodies react to highly stressful, traumatizing experiences is much more complex because of the influence of biologic, genetic, and social factors.

Another belief was that the actual structure of the brain remained relatively unaltered throughout aging. However, advanced imaging technology has changed all that. It has been clearly shown that not only are there significant changes in the size of the aging brain but these alterations also affect the key sites of our intellectual and emotional operating systems. At the same time there are also age-related changes in the endocrine and immune systems, both of which govern emotional responses.

AGEISM AS IT INFLUENCES DIAGNOSIS AND TREATMENT

There are many aspects of depression that are implicated as causes for its development. Scientists believe that some people inherit a biological structure that makes them more at risk for depression. Such a predisposition may have been passed from parents to children, or from even further down the lineage. But there are those individuals who become depressed for no easily identifiable reason.

All older adults experience medical conditions, bereavement, and changes in social supports. In time, most of them manage these transitions. While the ability to care for oneself is very closely linked to life satisfaction, overall health and well-being depends on what sense of control a person has over his own life. Being able to live in the setting of one's choice and having the desired degree of social support may offer protection from late-life depression to many elders.

Most elders and their families are not only unfamiliar with the symptoms of depression but they are also unaware that it is a medical illness. More important, they have no idea how or even *if* it should be treated. Unfortunately, there is still widespread acceptance of the well-entrenched myth that it is normal for elderly people to be depressed in the face of chronic illnesses, the loss of friends and spouses, and certain profoundly disruptive transitions such as no longer being able to drive or having to move out of one's home. Furthermore, there is an added taint of reproach from those who view depression as a character flaw or a personal failure. Caregivers and their loved ones may also feel a sense of shame. They often blame themselves for the illness and are too embarrassed to get help.

FACTORS THAT INCREASE THE RISKS FOR DEPRESSION

The major risk factors for depression include a personal or family history of depressive disorder, prior suicide attempts, female gender, lack of social supports, and current substance abuse. There is also a substantial social stigma surrounding depression that frequently prevents the best use of current knowledge and treatments.

Primarily, older women bear the greater risk since the evidence shows they are twice as likely as men to become seriously depressed. Not only do women live longer than men but biologic factors—chiefly hormonal influences—may be responsible for this susceptibility.

> Past or current depression in women is associated with decreased bone mineral density (Michaelson et al. 1996).

Other factors that contribute to the development of the disorder are:

- Most caregivers are women, and the stresses of maintaining relationships or caring for someone who is ill, especially a child or an elderly parent, appear to affect women more intensely.
- Those at risk include widowed or unmarried persons as well as anyone who lacks a supportive social network.
- Physical conditions such as heart disease, stroke, hip fractures, macular degeneration (a common type of vision impairment in the elderly), and some operative procedures, namely, bypass surgery, are known to be associated with the development of depression.

In general, clinicians and caregivers may suspect the disorder in an individual if recovery is delayed, treatments are refused, or if problems arise when the patient is being discharged from the hospital.

HOW COMMON IS DEPRESSION IN NURSING HOMES?

Large numbers of today's baby boomers, those born between 1946 and 1964, have loved ones who are living out their lives in nursing homes. This particular setting presents a very different state of circumstances for an older adult who is accustomed to living in his own home.

There is high prevalence of depression among today's 1.5 million nursing home residents. By definition, a nursing home admission confirms a person's loss of independence, sharply reduces his personal space, and virtually eliminates any possibility of privacy. Depression is a natural reaction to this formidable change of lifestyle. But even more important is the fact that depression often develops along with AD, Parkinson's, and other chronic diseases, all of which are well represented in any long-term care facility. Despite ample evidence of all these factors, many residents with depression will go untreated. These stricken individuals pay dearly in terms of pain and suffering.

There are several barriers to the identification and treatment of depression in long-term care, and some of the more prominent are:

- The complex features of both depression and dementia may make it difficult to distinguish one from the other.
- Insurance reimbursement and physicians' time constraints often hinder diagnosis and treatment.
- The number of trained personnel may be insufficient.

While healthcare workers have long suspected that depression is common among residents in long-term care, a 2006 study uncovered additional risk factors (Leonard 2006). The researchers revealed that depression triples the likelihood of a nursing home resident with dementia becoming physically aggressive. Furthermore, delusions, hallucinations, and constipation also appeared to be linked to hostile behavior. Although other studies have made associations between depression and physical aggression, no published study of treatment for this behavior mentioned medicating patients with antidepressants.

Threatening, intimidating behavior can be very traumatic for both residents and staff. All the contributing factors should be treated and modified. When a nursing home resident becomes disruptive that generally is a sign of an underlying condition. The behavior may be due to a urinary tract infection, pneumonia, or a need for toileting. Staff can be taught to assess the resident for these causes. Dementia is another contributor to aggression since memory loss leads to fear, increases disorientation, and exacerbates communication problems. Nursing home employees can also:

- Limit background distractions, such as a noisy TV or other activities that overwhelm the resident
- Redirect the attention of the disruptive resident
- Take vision and hearing deficits into consideration when talking to the resident
- Allow more time for the dementia patient to answer questions

If the intervention succeeds, the risks of violence and harm by afflicted residents may be significantly reduced (Leonard 2006).

Although many long-term care facilities have made depression screening a part of the admission process, in order to fully care for nursing home residents, *all* staff need more training in identifying the signs of depression. Family members need to their visit loved ones often and at different times of the day and in the evening, in order to closely monitor a facility's caregiving practices. They also should know what medications the resident is taking, why they are taking it, and what, if any, side effects have been noticed.

If a loved one is receiving a treatment, such as respiratory therapy or a dressing change, learn why it is needed and how effective it is.

It is generally true that depression resembles dementia—except for one consistent difference: residents with dementia will make an effort to answer a question, while depressed patients remain withdrawn, apathetic, and passive.

CAN DEPRESSION BE PREVENTED?

Individuals need to take an essential first step suggested for preserving good mental health, and that is to prepare for life's major changes. Two that readily come to mind are retirement and the possibility of moving out of the home one has lived in for many years. Additionally, there are other practical steps recommended for lowering the risk of depression:

- Cultivate, keep, and maintain friendships.
- Develop a hobby or learn a new skill. Have an interest that keeps both mind and body active.
- Keep in touch with family. Accept their help in times of sadness or loneliness.
- Stay fit by exercising and eating balanced, nutritious meals.
- Make the necessary lifestyle changes needed for good physical and mental health.

Identifying and treating an older adult's depression is just the beginning. Depression among older Americans should be screened for and treated no differently than other illnesses that become prevalent later in life, such as diabetes or high blood pressure.

As he informed the American public in his 1999 report on mental health, the US surgeon general Dr. David Satcher summed it up best when he concluded that mental illnesses such as depression are real and that treatment works. He encouraged families and caregivers to acknowledge the problem and get help. His advice can be summed up briefly: *Don't delay, act now!*

Chapter 5
Caregivers
Who Cares?

The number of people worldwide with dementia has been increasing at an alarming rate, keeping pace with the increase of our aging global population. It is estimated that 24.3 million people currently have dementia, with a projected 4.6 million new cases annually (Carillo and Milner 2005). These developments have triggered social issues never before seen on such a large scale. World leaders and healthcare officials have identified two major worries: the fear of overwhelming healthcare systems and the dread of having to depend on a dwindling working-age population for support (Lynn and Adamson 2003).

The aging population of baby boomers has the potential to overpower families and governments with a broad array of healthcare demands (Johnson and Wiener 2006).

Caregivers the world over share many of the same characteristics, responsibilities, and stresses. Typically, these caregivers are elderly spouses or adult children. The former have to deal with their own physical frailties, and the latter are holding jobs and maintaining their families as they meet the caring responsibilities. Most of them have assumed the caregiving role suddenly and with virtually no understanding of what this new responsibility entails. The issue of family caregiving is a vast and steadily growing problem that impinges on all aspects of daily life and ultimately will affect everyone in the community.

Demands on Caregivers

The price paid by caregivers is significant. The National Long-Term Care Survey (NIA, NIH 2006) and other research have documented that:

- Caregivers dedicate on average twenty hours per week to the provision of care for older persons and even more time when the older person has multiple disabilities;
- Caring for an older person with disabilities can be physically demanding, particularly for older caregivers who make up half of all caregivers. One-third of all caregivers describe their own health as fair to poor;
- Because caregiving is such an emotionally draining experience, caregivers have a high rate of depression when compared to the general population;
- Almost one-third of all caregivers is balancing employment and caregiving responsibilities, and of this group, two-thirds report conflicts in roles that require them to rearrange their work schedules, work fewer than normal hours, and/or take unpaid leaves of absence.

In the United States it is estimated that more than 6 million adults provide long-term, unpaid care to elderly members of their family (Tampi 2004). This seems difficult enough, but when an individual has dementia, which millions of elderly Americans do, the challenges are compounded. Seventy percent of people with Alzheimer's and other dementias live at home, cared for by family and friends (AA 2007). The economic aspects of home care combined with the physical and emotional demands of an AD patient adds exponentially to the burden (GAO 1994).

Although families have always taken care of their ill or impaired loved ones, present-day caregiving is not the same as it was a generation or two ago. It is much more difficult and challenging for the following reasons:

- The period of time for providing eldercare is much longer today.
- Today's care recipients are a good deal older and sicker.
- Because our society is much more mobile, often the care recipient lives a great distance from the primary caregiver.
- Most women are working outside of the home and are not readily available for caregiving.
- Working women often delay childbearing until their thirties and sometimes forties. They have young families at the same time their elderly parents need their help.

The long-term care of a family member can lead to exhaustion. It cannot be compared to caring for a child, because parents typically are optimistic for their child's future. When caring for an elderly family member whose condition is complicated by dementia, the burden steadily intensifies as the outlook is almost always bleak. As people live to older ages, the number of elders and burdened caregivers is expected to increase. Accordingly, this will create financial and human demands that will amount to a huge social liability.

Thoughtful planning is necessary for the most fundamental parental or spousal care arrangements. The common coping strategy of "taking one day at a time" may work for a while—as long as the circumstances remain stable and the changes are subtle.

For a variety of reasons it is more effective to work with a physician who has had experience with dementia patients. Finding someone with the knowledge and skills necessary to diagnose and treat the cognitively impaired can be reassuring and supportive for patients and families. Still, under the best circumstances, and despite paying

It took Lewis a long time to admit to himself that Margaret, his beloved wife of fifty-six years, had a serious problem. He arrived at that conclusion one morning after she woke up, turned to him and asked, "When are we going home?" She began following him around the house after that, asking the same question several times a day, for weeks. Additionally, he came to realize that she could no longer take care of herself. Margaret needed help with everything from brushing her teeth to eating her meals. Moreover, she was utterly lost in the kitchen, which she once had managed impeccably. However, Lewis rejected outright any family suggestions that Margaret should see a doctor. Nor would he seek outside help from any community resources. He was determined to handle the problem the way he always handled problems—by himself. After she wandered away from him when they were shopping together, his solution was to lock her in the house and do all the errands alone.

In Lewis's view, he alone was responsible for Margaret and he would be admitting weakness if he accepted any help from an outside source. Furthermore, as an intensely private person, he recoiled at the thought of exposing his life, his finances, or any other personal business to a community agency. But the worst feeling was that of impotence. Lewis felt powerless when faced with the changes he saw in someone he loved and lived with for so long.

careful attention to medical explanations and instructions, few individuals are able to repeat accurately "what the doctor said." Many physicians allow individuals to record what is said during the examination, but it is always best to ask in advance if a doctor's instructions can be tape recorded. Later it will be possible to play the tape for the family. Not only will they understand what transpired in the office, but it will be a good review for both patient and caregiver. Hearing the

Edie lived in the same town as her elderly parents. When her mother didn't return home from the hairdressers one afternoon, her frantic father called her at work. "She was supposed to call me so I could pick her up!" he shouted. Hours passed and finally a neighbor leaving a bank near the salon recognized the bewildered woman who was wandering aimlessly about the parking lot. She readily got into his car and he brought her to her home. Edie was appalled as her father berated his wife for wandering off, but after arguing for hours, she was able to convince him that her mother needed to see a physician. Edie's mother saw several specialists and submitted to much testing. She was diagnosed with a vascular dementia.

Edie's father was relieved. "At least it's not Alzheimer's," he said. Neither Edie nor her dad understood that the disease would advance and turn out to be just as destructive as AD.

tape played more than once will reinforce the doctor's comments and instructions. Furthermore, there will be no misunderstanding of the doctor's instructions between caregivers and families.

Great sensitivity to a patient's reaction is called for during a doctor's visit. Individuals with dementia will probably have more difficulty than most patients understanding all that a diagnosis entails. The doctor may even decide not to go into the finer points of the medical assessment. This is one of the times when there is no need to go into meticulous detail with the patient. The patient's reaction can be acknowledged and further explanations postponed. This is the time for reassurance of ongoing help and support rather than a clarification of the facts.

Doctors meet with patients alone and then with a family member or other advocate present. Individuals with dementia may have difficulty understanding all that their diagnosis entails but they certainly are entitled to know the significant facts. Healthcare professionals generally show great sensitivity toward all their patients and will acknowledge patients' reactions with sympathy and empathy. Questions are answered truthfully but care is taken not to overwhelm an elderly dementia patient by imparting more information than he or she can manage at the time. As a result, a physician may decide not to explain the complexities of medical assessment. For example, the doctor will not describe which areas of the brain govern memory or what physical alterations the brain has sustained. He will, however, tell the patient what imaging needs to be done, what medications may help, and kinds of other professionals who may be of assistance.

When someone has just received bad news it is important to explain the treatment plan, encourage questions, and reassure the individual that the staff will suggest resources for the patient and family as needed.

CAREGIVERS: CHALLENGES AND RESPONSIBILITIES

Sometimes it takes a cataclysmic event before a caregiver looks for specialized medical information or investigates the availability of community services. A loved one's unmanageable behavior or sudden reversal in health are two common examples. As soon as either event occurs, there is almost always a frantic effort to seek outside help. In the above case of Edie, the daughter of elderly parents, she would benefit by learning more about vascular dementia, also called multi-infarct dementia. She needs to know fully what dementia means and accept the responsibility of educating herself if her parents are unable to do so. Just looking up the word *dementia* would be a start.

The key issues apart from dementia are elders at risk—for instance, take Margaret and her husband, Lewis, from the above example. Margaret is at risk for injury either at the hands of her husband or as a result of wandering. Lewis is at risk for depression because he does not understand what stresses his wife's advancing dementia will cause, nor does he know there are agencies available to help him. Lewis could find out more by contacting a local Area

Agency on Aging (AAA). Margaret should have an intake evaluation done. After this a case worker will tell Lewis what their choices are. These will range from adult daycare and family counseling to homemaker services and in-home care.

When a dementia patient is living at home, caregivers and family members face a wide range of physical and emotional problems to cope with. There are constant, unrelenting, and stressful demands on their time, attention, and energy. Dealing with disruptive behavior, sleep disturbances, aggression, and agitation can be traumatic. It is a leading factor for institutionalization (Burke and Morgenlander 1999).

Fred lashes out because he has no insight into his illness, a common feature among individuals with dementia. He exhibits paranoid behavior and is likely to be depressed. During a comprehensive medical evaluation it was revealed that Fred had moderate AD, which meant that he had poor short-term memory and was beginning to lose his long-term memory. The examining clinician told Fred's sons about drug treatment,

Fred is a robust, sixty-eight-year-old widower whose two sons are worried about him. He has lived alone for several years since his wife died and always seemed to manage quite well. Lately, however, his appearance and demeanor are strikingly different, and for the past several weeks his sons have noticed some troubling behavior. Their father had been a successful business executive who was always well groomed and financially savvy. Now he seldom shaves, he is generally unkempt, and often discards his mail unread.

He has ample financial resources, yet he nearly lost his condo because of unpaid bills. When either of his sons offers to help with financial matters or even just to take him for a haircut, he becomes agitated. "They're trying to take over," and he claims they are "looking for trouble." It was only with great difficulty that they were able to take him to his doctor because at times he sounded threatening.

behavioral therapies, and physical and mental activities that have been shown to bring about improvement in some dementia patients. These include antipsychotic drugs for the paranoid behavior and antidepressant medication to help relieve depression. Behavioral therapy starts with counseling the caregiver, whether family member or professional, about the involuntary features of the patient's illness. Behavior can be modified more successfully when the caregiver learns to identify and eliminate the triggers of misconduct. For example, does the patient become aggressive and belligerent if he cannot find the bathroom or if there are several people talking to him at the same time? An environmental change may remove two triggers of inappropriate behavior. By limiting visitors and hanging a picture of a toilet on the bathroom door the family can encourage socially acceptable behavior.

Threatening behavior is often curbed by distracting and redirecting the patient. Music is soothing, as is stroking a pet. It is also important to maintaining a regular schedule for meals and toileting but to give a choice for an activity such as bathing (morning or evening). Daily, directed physical activities are always valuable because, in addition to improving and maintaining mobility, they serve as tension releases. Fred's doctor said that though some of Fred's conditions would not improve, at least by following the treatment plan, he could be better managed.

An essential element of the plan was to ensure that both the patient's family and the physician had a clear understanding about the behaviors being treated and the goals of treatment. Anything less would probably lead to unsatisfactory results (Burke and Morgenlander 1999). Fred's sons agreed to follow the physician's suggestions and were like-minded when faced with arranging for their father's home healthcare.

Many independent, community-dwelling older adults receive some type of assistance from family primarily because they have adult children nearby who help them, as did Fred. The 2002 Health and Retirement Study (HRS) indicates that about nine in ten older adults with disabilities have surviving adult children, and, despite the general assumption that most families are too scattered throughout the country to be able to help, 62.5 percent of elders have at least one adult child living within ten miles (Johnson and Wiener 2006).

Paid help is rare. Women, generally a spouse or daughter, tend to provide the bulk of unpaid informal care to impaired elders. However, providing help can easily overwhelm any caregiver, as mental health problems are extensive within the population of frail older adults.

The weight of caregiving responsibilities frequently creates significant stress for family helpers because the majority of them are also either working outside the home or struggling with their own health issues. The average age of these primary caregivers is about sixty years of age, and more than 75 percent from this group are women. Although there are many more devoted men who function as caregivers than there used to be, women are still in the majority. Clearly, caregiving is a women's issue (HHS 2005).

THE REALITY

Although most informal care is provided by one person, usually a daughter, many elders receive help from other people as well. Secondary caregivers generally are spouses and children of the primary caregiver, a son-in-law or a grandchild, for example. Although these individuals provide a wide variety of help, according to one study they do much less than the primary caregiver (Tennstedt 1999). Furthermore, when they do help, it is on an intermittent basis.

The burden of allocating tasks and assigning responsibilities weighs heavily on anyone with family obligations and it has obvious implications for tension and anxiety. Contributing to the turbulence is the fact that the primary caregiver often holds false expectations about the role the secondary caregiver should play. If assumptions are made as to "who does what" or if the details are vague and ambiguous, there surely will be problems. Another issue is disagreement among family members about the independence level of the individual in their care.

A common example is that of a relative viewing the patient as far more self-sufficient than the primary caregiver knows to be true.

Additional factors leading to differences of opinion occur when there are changes in caregiving conditions, usually when the patient's state of health worsens or when the primary caregiver's family or work requirements became more demanding (Usita, Hall, and Davis 2004).

Behavioral problems such as wandering and agitation have very powerful negative effects on the quality of life for families. At some point these behaviors occur in as many as 80 percent or more AD patients (Stewart 1995). There is a wide range of other behavioral problems inherent to dementia, such as sexually inappropriate conduct, violence, and anxiety (O'Brian, Shomphe, and Caro 2000). Agitated behavior can be nonaggressive, such as babbling, pacing, or repeating questions, or aggressive behavior such as screaming, kicking, or scratching.

These are just a few of the leading reasons for nursing home admission. However, whether a stricken individual is admitted due to unmanageable behavior or is already in a long-term care setting, families need to understand that institutionalization may be in the patient's best interest because more intensive care and supervision is necessary. It is surely more helpful to consider the act of placement as creating a resolution to a frustrating family situation rather than a crisis leading to nursing home admission. Above all, meeting the patient's needs is the primary concern.

THEIR OWN HOME OR A NURSING HOME?

"We've been married for fifty-three years and we married for better or for worse. I'm just honoring that contract!"

"I promised my mother many years ago that I would never put her in a nursing home."

"My father still lives alone, still drives, at age ninety-three. I'm proud of his independent attitude."

As noble as these sentiments may sound, there are some circumstances in which increased oversight or a more secure living situation might be a better choice. Quality of life is as important as length of life for many, and one's quality of life depends on, among other things, safe housing, adequate nutrition, emotional well-being, and appropriate healthcare services. Countless individuals have sincerely declared they would never put their elderly loved ones in a nursing home. Adult children, in particular, often feel they cannot break this promise. However, this is a promise most families simply cannot keep.

Aged spouses typically have their own health problems to deal with and even those in good health are rarely equipped, physically or emotionally, to fully care for an older adult who needs help with all the basic activities of daily living. It is simply not always possible to take care of a dementia patient at home for the duration of the disease. And, realistically, it can be a long, painful time of struggle before families finally agree the time has come for placement. Most caregivers initially underestimate the effects of increased stress; caregiving sometimes has unexpected adverse health consequences, including very high rates of depression. Thirty-two percent of caregivers reported six or more symptoms of depression and were classified as depressed (Covinsky et al. 2003).

Guilt, depression, and a sense of failure are common emotions faced by families who put a loved one in long-term care. The primary caregiver in particular usually consents to placement as a last resort when he or she feels overwhelmed, in a state of exhaustion and physically and emotionally depleted. However, the placement transition and the additional factors that affect caregiver health and well-being *after* placement of the patient have not been thoroughly investigated. A 2004 study shows that caregivers of dementia patients who must make the difficult decision to place their relatives into institutionalized care get no relief from depression and anxiety; in fact they often suffer additional emotional trauma following the decision (Schulz et al. 2004).

A four-year investigation coordinated by the University of Pittsburgh School of Medicine and led by Richard Schulz, PhD, director of

A sleep-deprived elderly man leans against the bedroom doorway as the early sunshine outlines the figure of his wife, asleep under the blanket. Thomas can barely keep his eyes open. His wife, Doris, diagnosed with Alzheimer's a few years ago, is starting to awaken and Thomas regards the moment with dread. He has learned how to get her to the bathroom, to get her dressed and fed, but there are other troubling behaviors he has not been able to manage.

Doris begins each day by asking him who he is and loudly demanding to know why he is in her room. Sometimes she accepts his explanation, but she often becomes tearful and anxious, convinced he is an intruder. She has attacked him twice and he was quite shaken when he found out how strong she was at the peak of her rage. He was also shocked to learn how quick he was to defend himself. Whenever he looks back on his wife's long struggle with the disease, he becomes discouraged and angry. He has tried so hard to manage this awful situation, yet he never feels he is gaining any ground. No matter what he does, there is no satisfaction, no sense of fulfillment.

Thomas is physically exhausted and he wonders how much longer he can continue to care for his beloved wife of forty-eight years. Each day is a day at war with her disease, and he has won very few battles. He loves her dearly, but he never dreamed of living with someone so totally dependent and vulnerable.

Although Thomas and his wife are childless, he is very close to his nephew. The nephew has often urged him to look into nursing home placement for Doris, but Thomas always rejected the suggestion because it made him feel a like failure. Now he is guilt-ridden and feels a powerful sense of shame. He finds himself thinking more and more about this as a distinct possibility.

the Center for Social and Urban Research at the university, determined that clinical intervention may greatly benefit caregivers by helping them prepare for the placement of their relatives and by treating their depression and anxiety during the placement process. "Caregivers who place their loved ones in an institution do not get the sense of relief or experience the closure observed among caregivers whose loved ones pass away," said Dr. Schulz. "They continue to feel distressed because of the suffering and decline of their loved one as well as having to face new challenges such as frequent trips to the long-term facility, reduced control over the care provided their relative, and taking on responsibilities such as coordinating and monitoring care," he added. Researchers recommended treating caregivers' emotional distress through or by enhanced counseling and support group meetings, educating them about the nature of long-term care facilities and their impact on patient functioning, engaging them in end-of-life planning, and preparing them for the eventual death of their family member.

There are also many overlooked and underserved elders who expend great efforts to maintain their independence by living alone. However, all too often the cost of this independence turns out to be social isolation. As the senior population of the United States swells, and as the popular movement to assist elderly people to "age in place" gathers momentum, the issue of senior isolation becomes increasingly important.

Aging in place refers to residing in a dwelling that an individual has called home for many years. It refers to living in a nonhealthcare environment and using services that allow the individual to remain at home even when circumstances change.

As the elderly population grows and subsequently triggers the need for adequate elderly health and housing services, the resources to provide services will decrease. Medicare already funds healthcare at levels the federal government cannot afford much longer. The trustees of the Medicare Trust Fund have warned that the healthcare program for the elderly and disabled faces insolvency by the year 2020. The improvement in medical science has extended the life span of our elderly population, thus extending the number of years the elderly will utilize Medicare. Finding a more efficient means of service delivery is of paramount importance. However, the current connections between elderly health and housing are questionable at best. As a result, the most desirable and most cost-efficient method of growing old, aging in place, is difficult, even under the most ideal conditions.

There is ample evidence showing that loneliness is linked to both physical and mental health problems. Some of the added risks older adults living alone are exposed to are malnutrition, dehydration, infections, miscellaneous physical injuries, and falls. By some estimates, each year approximately a quarter of all older adults sustain at least one fall. More important, half the time the person who falls is unable to get up. And, regrettably, it is not uncommon for elderly people living alone to be found helpless or even dead in their own homes (Yeh and Lo 2004).

If the goal is for older adults to avoid premature hospitalization and subsequent institutionalization, then the importance of social, physical, and emotional support from others needs much more emphasis. It is essential that increasing the social support and facilitating of friendships be factored into lifestyle management for communities of elderly persons. On the surface, the idea of older adults who can live independently may seem to be a worthy aspiration. Still, since all of us depend more on others as we age, more attention needs to be paid to the concept and practice of interdependence in order to avoid social isolation.

HOME MODIFICATION

Before taking steps to bring professional help into the home or to move a frail elder into a more protective setting, some families adapt the home to meet the elder's needs. Home modifications and repairs can improve safety, ease the way older adults perform daily activities such as bathing, cooking, and climbing stairs, as well as maintain the value of the home.

Home modifications customize living spaces for people with physical limitations so that they can continue to live independently and safely. Such modifications range from the simple fixes, such as getting rid of scatter rugs or fitting doors with more comfortable door handles for elders who usually have arthritic fingers. There are also sensors available that will help open doors, which are a totally different product from the safety sensors installed to prevent wandering. Of course there are more complex additions like installing an electric stair lift. Depending on the situation, some homes may need minimal conversion while others require full-scale construction projects for widening doorways or installing a wheelchair ramp.

The main benefit of making home modifications is that they promote independence and help to prevent accidents. Eighty-two percent of older Americans prefer to stay where they are as long as possible. A nationwide telephone survey of two thousand midlife and older Americans conducted in November/December 1999 (Bayer and Harper 2000) also found that

- 70 percent of those able to make changes have made at least one modification to make their homes easier to live in;
- 85 percent have made simple changes to their homes; and
- 67 percent of those making changes believe doing so will allow them to live there longer than they would have otherwise been able to. The general estimate was that these changes would allow for another ten or more years.

Most housing is designed for younger, more active, and more mobile people. To live at home, a person must have access to transportation and shopping and be able to do household chores. Many older adults will lose one or more of these abilities as they age.

Research by the Centers for Disease Control and Prevention shows that home modifications and repairs may prevent 30 to 50 percent of all home accidents among seniors, including falls (Bayer and Harper 2000).

Common Examples of Home Modifications

- Grab bars in the bathroom, including by the bathtub, shower, and toilet
- Handheld flexible shower heads
- Handrails on both sides of staircases and for outside steps
- Lever-operated faucets that are easy to turn on and off
- Sliding or revolving shelves for cabinets in the kitchen

As expected, the cost of such projects is a fundamental concern. Many minor home modifications and repairs can be done for about $150 to $2,000. For bigger projects, some financing options may be available. For instance, many home-remodeling contractors offer reduced rates and charge sliding-scale fees based on a senior's income and ability to pay. Another suggestion is that the homeowner try to obtain a modest loan to cover urgent needs. Other possible sources of public and private financial assistance include the following.

- Title III of the Older Americans Act provides for home modification and repair funds that are to be distributed by the local department of elder affairs or Area Agency on Aging (AAA). To contact a local AAA anywhere in the United States, call the US Administration on Aging's Eldercare Locator at 1-800-677-1116 or visit the Eldercare Locator Web site at http://www.eldercare.gov.
- Rebuilding Together, Inc., a national volunteer organization, is able to assist some low-income seniors through its local affiliates with home modification efforts. More information is available by contacting a local Area Agency on Aging, or Rebuilding Together at 1-800-4-REHAB-9 or http://www.rebuildingtogether.org.
- Investment capital is offered by the US Department of Energy's Low-Income Home Energy Assistance Program (LIHEAP) and

the Weatherization Assistance Program (WAP). Both of these programs are run by local energy and social services departments. For example, Tennessee residents would go to http://www.tennessee.gov/humanserv/adfam/afs_w.htm. For LIHEAP, go to http://www.acf.hhs.gov/programs/ocs/liheap.

- A reverse mortgage is a unique type of home loan that permits a homeowner to convert the equity in his or her home into cash. It can give older Americans more financial reserves with which to supplement Social Security, meet unexpected medical expenses, or make home improvements. For more information visit the Housing and Urban Development (HUD) Web site at http://www.hud.gov/buying/rvrsmort.cfm. A reverse mortgage is not for everyone. It is important that homeowners fully understand the prospective benefits, financial risks, and other potential pitfalls to ensure that they make informed choices.

If you are aware of fraud, waste, and abuse in HUD programs and operations, report it to HUD's Inspector General Hotline at:

Toll free 1-800-347-3735
TDD 202-708-2451

Or write to:

Department of Housing and Urban Development
Office of Inspector General Hotline
Assistant Inspector General for Investigations
451 7th Street, SW, Room 8270
Washington, DC, 20410

Karen, fifty-one, had always been concerned about her eighty-eight-year-old mother, Milly, who had been living alone for several years. When she answered a frantic phone call from her mother's neighbor in the Florida retirement complex where both elderly women lived, Karen knew that the time had come to bring Milly back north and help her move into an assisted-living setting. From the call she learned Milly seldom changed her clothes, couldn't manage her medications, and had numerous minor car accidents. The neighbor also told Karen there was an incident when her mother was unable to get out of the bathtub and the fire department was called to rescue the hysterical old lady. Clearly the decision could no longer be postponed.

In the beginning, Milly accepted the plan enthusiastically; what could be better than to be closer to her family? The residence she moved to was new and attractive, the employees were friendly and helpful, and now she would see much more of her only child and her beloved grandchildren.

The "sandwich generation" represents those who not only care for their own children but also act as caregivers for their own parents. Up to 40 percent of caregivers belong to this growing segment of the population, caring for children under eighteen in addition to other family members (Young 2002). Karen is a new member since she only recently assumed her eldercare responsibilities. She feels caught between the often conflicting demands of her own family and her elderly mother. Her life is now particularly stressful and hectic, and this is affecting her work. Even if she cannot change her mother's behavior, she needs to alter her own.

One strategy Karen could use is screening her calls at work and home. The phone calls may decrease if she mounts a large calendar near her mother's telephone and notes the days she and her husband will visit or phone. She also needs to get her family together and dis-

Karen breathed a sigh of relief. No longer was her mother hundreds of miles away, a menace on the road and missing her medications. Karen's husband was very supportive and insisted on visiting his mother-in-law frequently to see if she needed anything. Best of all, Karen's teenaged son offered to help by driving his grandmother to the doctor's and hairdresser's and other appointments. Karen smiled to herself—with all this help, she felt for sure things were going to work out very well indeed!

Initially, the changeover from the retirement complex to the assisted-living setting was without incident, but before long there were problems. For example, Karen hadn't anticipated being called at home and work several times a day and having to listen to the same whining, repetitive harangue. Her mother complained about not being able to drive and threatened to leave her new apartment and to return to Florida. Furthermore, Karen was shocked to hear her own son criticize her for letting his grandmother live anywhere without her own car. He thinks she is fine and perfectly capable of driving.

cuss, once again, the reasons for Milly's move. As the primary caregiver, Karen also needs to clarify caregiving and household responsibilities for each family member and needs to warn all of them about unrealistic expectations. Most assisted-living settings sponsor support groups, but if Karen cannot attend a group meeting she can participate in one of the many chat rooms and message boards available online. A good place to start is at http://www.alz.org/living_with_alzheimers _message_boards_lwa.asp.

There are those who manage their caregiving responsibilities with just a few minor adjustments in their daily routines. After some fine-tuning of their schedules they are able to fulfill caregiving obligations and discover that the satisfaction they experience from helping a loved one has its own rewards. Others discover that looking after someone is done at not only great personal expense, but that there are unanticipated professional sacrifices as well, as studies in family caregiving have revealed. Additionally, a sizeable number of caregivers find their work, mental health, and personal relationships are noticeably affected. New caregivers quickly learn that integrating caregiving with work-related obligations is not only far more difficult than they could ever have imagined, but that it can have adverse and long-term professional effects. In retrospect, few expected it would be necessary to turn down career opportunities. Others are dismayed to find they are overlooked for career advancement. The results of an in-depth study of fifty-five caregivers who had made some type of work adjustment as the result of their caregiving responsibilities revealed that the average lifetime financial loss was estimated at more than $659,000 in lost wages, Social Security benefits, and retirement contributions (MMMI 1999).

Most working caregivers struggle constantly to make scheduling and other workplace modifications in order to create a feasible balance. As an example, a recent study noted that one of the most frequent adjustments is to change the time coming to or leaving the workplace. It follows, however, that workers who defer promotions, take leaves of absence, or refuse to relocate or to travel because they are taking care of a loved one pay a significant price. They will earn less during their working life and consequently will have reduced retirement benefits (Wagner 2003).

The growing elderly population and the caregiving they require from their families should sound a warning to business. Employers reported a 72 percent increase in staffing-related problems due to caregiving since 1990, and more than 40 percent of them report they have no plan in place to assist caregivers in this growing dilemma (HRI 2000).

To be fair, employers are not always aware of the caregiving issues their employees are dealing with. Caring for an older adult is a sensitive and often confidential subject for employees, who are often hesitant to share their concerns with employers. The privacy issue may be the primary reason why eldercare issues are usually not discussed in the workplace. Everyone is familiar with parental leave and daycare for children, but the needs of an employee who is caring for an aging relative are seldom known. Programs to assist working caregivers continue to lag behind programs for childcare (Neal and Wagner 2001). As an example, many employers do not know about workers who must travel extensively to handle the long-distance care of a family member. Furthermore, eldercare is not limited to parents and older relatives, but often refers to one spouse taking care of the other.

Given that these challenges are unique, it can be difficult for employers to fully understand their workers' caregiving responsibilities. As employee issues in this area expand and become increasingly complex, businesses will be faced with the consequences of an aging population dependent on working caregivers.

As previously mentioned, one option is to get in touch with an Area Agency on Aging (AAA). With the passage of the National Family Caregiver Support Program in 2000, all AAAs are mandated to address the needs of family caregivers. Respite care (the patient goes to a nursing home or other location for a brief period of time to give the caregiver an interval of relief), additional in-home help, and referral to adult daycare are some examples. When an AAA works together with area employers, the chances for excellent and cost-effective ways to reach out to caregivers are distinctly improved (Wagner 2003).

Typically, businesses that offer supportive policies are beneficial because employees are more productive. Additional positive outcomes are job satisfaction, employee loyalty, less turnover, and less intrusion of professional obligations into family life. It is not unusual for major organizations and businesses to be slow in recognizing the tremendous cost and productivity drains on employers caused by workers who are burdened with caregiving issues. An online survey of 140 executives nationwide by the Boston-based human resources consulting firm Veritude found eldercare was ranked last in a list of considerations as a component for an ideal workplace (Jackson 2005). AARP CEO William D. Novelli said at a forum that more than one-third of US workers are providing eldercare (Yandrick 2001).

Employees subject to the demands of caregiving unknowingly add stress to the workplace, reduce productivity, and accelerate turnover.

Furthermore, the business sector needs to understand that as the population of older adults increases, more workers will be thrust into managing eldercare issues. Therefore, a practical tactic is to develop formal policies on eldercare. The place to start is with human resource personnel who are well positioned to develop timely strategies for employees to learn what eldercare referral services are available and how to access them. During the White House Conference on Aging in 2005, the number-one problem identified was the fact that caregivers do not know where to start to find resources. Officials overwhelmingly agreed that one solution would be to create a comprehensive hotline where all services would be available to assist caregivers. Preparing now offers businesses competitive advantages in terms of productivity, retention, and bottom-line results.

In 2006 the Family Caregiver Alliance's National Center on Caregiving released a new issue brief on the value of paid family and medical leave for both working families and employers. A law to this effect is already in place in California and other states are soon to follow (FCA 2006).

SHARPENING HEALTH LITERACY SKILLS

Whether a patient or a caregiver, anyone without training in a health-related area can easily misunderstand a doctor's orders. Even well-educated people with strong reading and writing skills may have trouble understanding a medical document or a doctor's instructions regarding a drug or a procedure. Furthermore, irrespective of educational background, managing the masses of paperwork generated by a person's medical care and treatment can be overwhelming.

The Institute of Medicine (IOM) defines *health literacy* as "the degree to which individuals can obtain, process, and understand the basic information and services they need to make appropriate health decisions." Evidence indicates that an astonishing 90 million Americans have misunderstood in whole or in part what their doctors have said about their diagnosis and treatment (IOM 2004). Knowledge gaps range from having an unclear view about a loved one's diagnosis to taking medicine incorrectly or misunderstanding insurance forms.

Inadequate health literacy is linked to a tendency to skip preventive care, a habit that increases risks for noncompliance, treatment failure, and unnecessary hospitalization. Individuals bear responsibility for their health status: adopting a healthy lifestyle and participating in risk prevention programs are two ways to maintain physical well-being. Although reading, writing, and math skills are part of maintaining basic health literacy, patients also need to know how to listen and ask relevant questions in order to acquire helpful feedback concerning their condition.

It is essential to know how to advocate for oneself or for a family member who is unable to do so. In order to prepare the way for developing one's advocacy abilities, the Partnership for Clear Health Communication (available online at http://www.askme3.org/PFCHC) created the "Ask Me 3" educational program. Although many people do go to the doctor's office with a list of pertinent questions, they may not include the most direct and effective. The "Ask Me 3" plan consists of three concise questions designed to improve discussion between patient and doctor regarding the reason for the visit. They are:

1. What is my main problem?
2. What do I need to do?
3. Why is it important for me to do this?

All consumers are urged to ask these questions when seeing a doctor, dentist, or pharmacist or preparing for a medical test or procedure.

If all doctor's visits were conducted in a comfortable, welcoming atmosphere devoid of time pressure and if every patient was encouraged to question anything unclear, outcomes might have a better chance of being more mutually satisfactory. Patients who understand what they are being told are more likely to follow directions consistently and, consequently, see more favorable results.

How to Improve Your Health Literacy

- Click on www.askme3.org for worksheets to use when seeing a physician.
- Prepare a list of questions before keeping an appointment.
- Be sure you understand what the doctor is talking about.
- Ask for written information to take home and review.
- Talk to the physician about your questions and concerns when fully dressed, not when wearing a hospital gown and sitting on an examining table.

Patients with low health literacy typically have difficulty understanding the names of prescription medications, why they need to take them, and dosing instructions. This confusion leads to missed doses or doses taken at the wrong time. It also can lead to a disconnect between what the patient and doctor think the patient is taking. When the doctor and patient agree on what drugs the patient is taking, there is less likelihood of medication errors and adverse effects.

Benefits Checkup

The Benefits Checkup is an online service designed to screen for federal, state, and some local private and public benefits for adults fifty-five and older, available online at www.benefitscheckup.org. The site also provides a service called BenefitsCheckupRx that identifies public and private programs that can help pay for prescription drugs. It is the first and only Web-based service that offers older adults a personalized report of prescription savings they otherwise may not have known they were eligible to receive.

WHO IS A CAREGIVER AND WHERE IS THE HELP?

Anyone who is concerned about the safety and well-being of an aging relative or friend and helps that individual with their household tasks, for example, bill paying, grocery shopping, or personal care, is a caregiver. However, the word *caregiver* was not used in previous generations. Families simply took care of their disabled or frail elderly members as a matter of course. Again, women did not customarily work outside the home in previous generations, nor did the elderly live as long as they now do. If any supplementary help was available, it was informal and typically turned out to be another family member. There were no official government programs or community agencies as we know them today.

An often overlooked barrier to seeking resources is the perception some people have about what constitutes a caregiver. There are many who fit the description yet do not see themselves in this light. Or if they do, they seldom realize that there may be help readily available in their own community.

Although families and friends traditionally have provided the necessary assistance for elderly loved ones to remain in their homes and communities, they face ever-increasing demands on their limited time and other resources. Most family caregivers find that providing care to their loved ones is greatly rewarding. Nonetheless, balancing careers, the needs of other family members, and personal needs with the complexities of caring for frail and sometimes cognitively impaired older persons can be a heavy burden. The majority of family caregivers (79 percent) are providing care to someone over the age of fifty (MMMI 2006). However, few families can do it all without outside help.

Very few individuals are prepared to be caregivers, one of the most challenging responsibilities of a lifetime. Most will need assistance. The Older Americans Act, signed into law by President Lyndon Johnson in 1965, created the basic framework for organizing, coordinating, and providing community-based services and opportunities for older Americans and their families. The act as amended in 2000 contains an important new program, the National Family Caregiver Support Program (NFCSP), the purpose of which is to help the hundreds of thousands of family caregivers responsible for ill elderly or disabled relatives (AoA 2004). The program was developed by the Administration on Aging, an agency of the US Department of Health and Human Services. State agencies on aging work with Area Agencies on Aging (AAAs) and community and service organizations to provide support services. These services include:

- Giving information to caregivers about supplemental services that complement the care provided by families
- Assistance to caregivers in gaining access to the services
- Individual counseling
- Organized, professionally facilitated support groups
- Caregiver training to assist families in making decisions and solving problems about their caregiving roles
- Respite care to provide temporary relief for caregivers from their responsibilities

Caregivers can familiarize themselves with the eldercare agencies listed in the city or county government sections of the telephone directory under aging or social services. It may take some time to analyze the resources and learn what best meets an individual's needs, but it is reassuring to learn that assistance exists.

The Alzheimer's Association has launched a comprehensive Web site called Carefinder (www.alz.org/carefinder), which gives information on such topics as planning ahead, care options, coordinating care, and support. By using the questionnaire on this site, individuals can get a useful report that is tailored to their specific needs in several ways. It includes questions to ask healthcare providers, care recommendations, and even suggestions for seldom anticipated future problems. Furthermore, the care recipient need not have Alzheimer's since the information provided is applicable to caregivers dealing with a wide range of chronic illnesses. Another resource for caregivers is found at AARP's new Navigating the World of Caregiving site at www.aarp.org/caregivers. Contents includes interactive tools, worksheets, articles, and videos.

GENDER DIFFERENCES

The caregiver profile in the United States has changed. Once predominantly female, there has been a sizeable increase in the number of men involved. The National Family Caregivers Association reports that men make up approximately 44 percent of the nation's caregivers (NFCA 2000).

Regardless of the illness their loved one may have, male caregivers readily acknowledge that the responsibility is stressful and all-consuming. Men, however, are not intimidated by this nontraditional role even though they acknowledge that some of the tasks may seem to be outside their comfort zone. They seem to approach the business of caregiving pragmatically. Men have a tendency to assess caregiving situations differently than women in the sense that men apply problem-solving techniques as they might in a workplace setting. For example, men display less hesitation in bringing in outside help when confronted with some of the aspects of care. They appear to be less reticent in delegating tasks and more willing to call social workers and contact healthcare agencies when faced with problems that require professional solutions. Men also willingly admit they need help when circumstances are beyond their skill level and make it a point to learn what needs to be done. They either decide to do it themselves or authorize someone else to do it. Men are getting the job done and in greater numbers than ever before.

There is, however, one caregiving area in which women overshadow men. Despite the fact that support groups have been shown to ease anxiety and reduce the social isolation that accompanies caregiving, men lag behind women in their readiness to participate in such groups (Trubo 2002).

LONG-DISTANCE CAREGIVING

Providing care for an elderly relative comes in many forms. Some caregivers live near their family members and are "hands-on" participants, while others are many miles away and manage care from afar. Long-distance caregiving can be just as stressful, or even more so, than being on site because all the routine and expected worries are magnified when a caregiver is far away.

There was a time when the situation Antoinette now manages was the norm. However, social changes have affected most families, and parents no longer expect their adult children will live in close proximity—or even live in the same state. Millions of people are long-distance caregivers who are faced with situations like Ted's. They spend their time finding and coordinating health professionals and services while dealing with the care recipients. Distance caregivers assume the responsibility of organizing family members and suggesting assignments. They remain as involved as they possibly can in protecting their loved one's health and well-being and can be highly effective no matter how great the distance.

Long-distance caregiving goes far beyond e-mails, phone calls, or lengthy discussions about symptoms, insurance forms, and prescription coverage. It also entails much more than a semi-annual site visit, although every visit is significant for both safety and social reasons. For example, a visit can be an opportunity to determine if the care recipient has an advance directive indicating healthcare treatment preferences (see chapter 8) and for recording lists of medicines,

Antoinette is a young widow sharing a two-family house with her parents. She lives upstairs and they occupy the first floor. Her father is a newly diagnosed diabetic, and before he was discharged from the hospital she learned how to test his blood sugar and give him insulin injections. Her mother is legally blind. Antoinette monitors her father's diabetes, helps her mother, and takes care of her own three small children.

Ted lives four hundred miles away from his seventy-plus-year-old parents who recently moved into senior housing in a mid-sized city. His younger brother is in the armed forces, stationed overseas. Since the move, Ted has been very involved in helping his folks understand their new health insurance forms, searching for medical information for them, and helping them pay their bills. His mother is fairly comfortable using a computer and much of this has been done online. Their usual social phone calls alternate with informative e-mails, and when he speaks with either parent, they can all simultaneously look at the same form or bill as he explains it. Ted sees them every few months and the next time he visits, he plans to install a webcam and show them how it works.

names, and phone numbers of the prescribing doctors. A long-distance caregiver also needs to get to know a trusted neighbor, friend, or clergy member and ask to be called immediately in case of a crisis. Paying a personal call is the surest way to assess an individual's living quarters for warning signs such as an accumulation of clutter, unopened mail, poor lighting, spoiled or scarcity of food in the refrigerator, weight loss, neglected hygiene, the absence of grab bars in the bathroom, and loose rugs or wiring.

Long-distance caregiving presents special challenges, and some families choose to employ a professional to help manage day-to-day supervision of a loved one. In the private sector, a geriatric care manager (GCM) serves as a consultant for families with dependent older adults or as a contracted agent representative for corporate employees' benefit services. Geriatric care managers are professionals who specialize in helping older people and their families with long-term care arrangements. They often have training in gerontology, social work, nursing, or counseling, and also have extensive knowledge about the cost, quality, and availability of services in an older person's community. Consequently, geriatric care managers can help:

- Conduct care-planning assessments to identify problems and determine eligibility for assistance and the need for services
- Screen, arrange, and monitor in-home help
- Review financial, legal, or medical issues and offer referrals to geriatric healthcare professionals to conserve assets and maintain good health and well-being
- Solve safety issues and provide crisis intervention
- Act as a liaison to families living away from the parent, making sure things are going well and alerting families to problems
- Help move an older person to or from a retirement complex, nursing home, or other residence
- Provide consumer education and advocacy
- Offer counseling and support

Before deciding to hire a professional of this type, it is important to make sure that such a specialist needs to be involved. If families are ambivalent about eldercare, it is worthwhile to discuss the situation fully with a physician, social worker, clergy member, or trusted friend to clarify the potential care recipient's needs.

The field of geriatric care management is not strictly regulated, and many people with specialized training identify themselves as care managers. While there are no licensing requirements for GCMs, there are certification programs. Determine if a candidate is certified and from where.

It is beneficial and practical to enlist the support of other family members when planning to consult a professional because this is a good way to build a consensus on the solutions. Questions that you may want to ask a GCM are:

- How long have you been working in this field?
- How are after-hours emergencies handled?
- Should we work with more than one geriatric care manager?
- What are your rates and do you have references?
- Do you have a copy of your professional standards of practice?

Such a document provides information on fiduciary responsibilities and privacy concerns.

Sources for Finding Geriatric Care Managers

- Area Agencies on Aging/Departments of Elder Affairs
- Hospitals, senior centers, geriatric assessment centers, and charitable organizations, such as the Alzheimer's Association
- The National Association of Professional Geriatric Care Managers at (520) 881-8008
- The Eldercare Locator Service at (800) 677-1116

Organizations That Promote Standards for Geriatric Care Managers Include

National Association of Professional Geriatric Care Managers
1604 North Country Club Road
Tucson, AZ 85716
(520) 881-8008; fax (520) 325-7925

National Council on Aging
409 Third Street, SW
Suite 200
Washington, DC 20024
(202) 479-1200; fax (202) 479-0735

Case Management Society of America
8201 Cantrell Road
Suite 230
Little Rock, AR 72227
(501) 225-2229; fax (501) 221-9068

ALTERNATIVE LIVING SITUATIONS/ COMMUNITY RESOURCES

There is a persistent myth that most of our nation's elderly live in nursing homes. The truth is that only about 5 percent live in a long-term care setting and many frail elderly, even in advanced old age, can comfortably live independently as long as they have the necessary support (Samarrai 2002). There are a variety of community agencies offering a selection of services to make this possible.

Not to be overlooked is the opportunity to use these services even if the elder prefers an alternative-living arrangement such as congregate housing or assisted living. By maximizing community resources, many frail physically impaired older adults are able to continue to live on their own in safety and comfort.

Some alternative-living situations frail elders have chosen include:

• Moving into the caregiver's home
• Living in a board and care home
• Living in adult foster care
• Congregate housing
• Life care or continuing care in a retirement community
• Sharing their home
• Residing in a long-term care setting

Communities throughout the United States offer a wide variety of services for their aging populations. Use the Eldercare Locator as the first step to learn about services in your loved one's community. Some of the better-known public organizations are

• Senior centers, which offer older people an opportunity to meet and socialize. They offer a wide variety of social, educational, and recreational programs. Some senior centers provide transportation services and lunch.
• Adult daycare, agencies that provide a variety of health and

social services to elders who need help with personal care and other activities of daily living. Adult daycare not only provides respite for family caregivers but it is also a convenient location for some types of therapeutic care for cognitively and physically impaired older adults. This setting has allowed many caregivers the option to continue working while the client is safe, cared for, and able to participate in socializing with peers and receiving needed therapies.

- Area Agencies on Aging (AAAs). The Administration on Aging awards funds mandated by the Older Americans Act (OAA) to State Units on Aging (SUA), which are located in every state.

Chapter 6
Dementia
Facts and Fiction

Myths about dementia abound. One of the most persistent, widespread, and potentially dangerous myths about senility equates dementia with normal aging. *Senility* stems from *senilis*, the Latin word for old, and it pertains to the mental or physical weaknesses associated with old age. It has long been paired with dementia, and the term *senile dementia* was once standard medical terminology, regularly used when diagnosing any confused older adult. Senility and senile dementia are lesser-used terms that support the belief that cognitive impairment is to be expected as a person ages. This myth is extremely dangerous when held by health professionals. It can lead to a lack of prevention and treatment measures, thus becoming a self-fulfilling prophecy. If families are simply told to anticipate forgetting, confusion, poor judgment, and personality changes in their elderly loved one because it is typical in old age, there may be no further professional assessment of the individual, let alone treatment options.

FACTS ABOUT DEMENTIA

Dementia is not a normal factor in the aging process; it is a severe form of cognitive and intellectual deterioration. It is not the name of a specific disease but rather a word used to describe the mental condition of someone whose memory is impaired and whose problems with processing information are severe enough to impair normal functioning. The first symptom of the disorder is usually memory loss. Most dementias are serious irreversible diseases, but a number of them can be reversed when treated appropriately.

There are a variety of causes of dementia. Depression, malnutrition, dehydration, and drug interactions can all lead to dementia. Depression can appear to be dementia but can be treated with talk therapy or medication, and very often the cognitive impairments mistaken for dementia will be reversed when the depression is treated. Malnutrition can affect cognition; however, once the person receives proper nutrition and is well hydrated, often the dementia lifts. Furthermore, many clinicians are convinced that the most common of all cognitive problems are those triggered by drug interactions. Physicians always need to be accurately informed of all medications an individual is taking, both prescription and nonprescription. It is the only way to avoid effects that are at best unpleasant, at worst life-threatening.

Organic brain syndrome is a general name given to a variety of mental deficits found in elders that are not psychiatric in origin but rather are caused by physical disorders. However, organic brain syndrome, senility, and senile dementia are imprecise terms.

The assumption that once a person reaches sixty-five certain intellectual functions such as thinking, remembering, and decision making will inevitably deteriorate can have dangerous consequences. Individuals who believe that cognitive decline is a normal feature of growing old will either ignore significant symptoms or make health decisions based on incorrect or outdated information. And, although normal aging is characterized by slower recall of information and a longer processing time for new data, neither is related to dementia. Nevertheless, many elderly and their families believe the senility myth and suffer the unfortunate consequences.

Most older Americans cope successfully with the customary physical and cognitive changes associated with aging. They also deal with retirement, changes in lifestyle, as well as the wrenching losses of family members and friends. However, a substantial proportion of the population aged fifty-five years and older, which is roughly 20 percent, experience mental disorders that are not part of normal aging. The most common disorders, in order of prevalence, are anxiety, severe cognitive impairment including AD, and mood disorders. These disorders can be debilitating and severely affect an older adult's quality of life (AAGP 2004).

Negative myths and stereotypes are at the heart of age discrimination. A particularly detrimental fiction is that elderly persons cannot process new information. Older people are often portrayed as frail, tired, self-pitying, dull, unhappy, intolerant, and unproductive. However, historically there have always been elderly individuals who were models of leadership, management, and creativity throughout the ages. As examples, Konrad Adenauer's political career in Germany spanned sixty years. He is best known as chancellor of West Germany from 1949 to 1963, the oldest in German history. Arthur Rubinstein, one of the greatest pianists of the twentieth century, performed concerts internationally until he was eighty-nine. Barbara Cartland, who holds the *Guinness Book of World Records* title for most published author, wrote well into her nineties. Other far less prominent older adults have achieved success after sixty in countless other endeavors.

Ideally, every older adult should be respected as a resourceful, valued member of society, capable of much more if encouraged to develop his potential or contribute his wisdom and abilities. But sustaining healthy cognitive functioning as people age is not guaranteed. As illustrated in the Seattle Longitudinal Study, it depends on several factors: continued cognitive activity, a healthy body, a positive state of mind, physical exercise, and a supportive social environment (Schaie 2005).

Rose is a lonely widow who lives in the same neighborhood she moved to as a newlywed. Despite many changes over the years, Rose was always comfortable in her small apartment and she saw no reason to move. The market was just a few blocks away, and she easily managed to walk to church on Sunday and her hairdressers for weekly appointments.

Rose enjoyed weekly visits from her son, who lived nearby. Then, abruptly, he was transferred to another state and for almost four months did not see his mother. He relied on frequent phone calls to keep in touch. Gradually, he began to develop uneasy feelings after those calls; his mother's voice was toneless and almost monosyllabic.

Impulsively, he flew home one weekend and surprised her. When she answered the door he was shocked. His mother, who was always slender and attractive, now appeared gaunt and unkempt. He saw clutter everywhere: newspapers scattered, dirty dishes covering the kitchen table, several weeks' worth of unopened mail. Peering into the refrigerator he found only a container of milk, half a loaf of stale bread, and some outdated medications. The freezer held four identical frozen dinners. Rose looked her son blankly and told him she was not hungry, just a little tired.

When she was examined by a physician, Rose could tell him who she was but she could not answer other routine, simple questions. She also could not follow simple commands such as "close your eyes" and "raise your right hand." At this point, her son was sure she had Alzheimer's disease.

But a careful review of her prescriptions revealed that confusion and fatigue were common side effects of two of her medications. She was also seriously dehydrated, malnourished, and mildly depressed. This patient responded well to treatment for her dehydration, malnutrition, and depression. She also became much more alert and better oriented after her drug regimen was modified.

WHAT IS MEANT BY GOOD BRAIN HEALTH
AND HOW CAN YOU ACHIEVE IT?

Ask any health professional what is meant by good brain health and you will get a wide variety of answers, but they will all agree on the same general premise: a healthy brain is one that functions at optimum capacity with little if any impairment of mental activities. It operates normally, governing all the body's systems, thereby fulfilling its purpose.

There are several ways to maintain brain health. Mental stimulation and lifelong learning can help avoid or delay the onset of memory loss and cognitive deficits in later life. Some experts point to the influence of lifelong education and recommend taking a course or developing a skill, such as learning a new language or how to use a computer. Others extol the merits of word games, chess, reading, and discussion groups.

Paul Nussbaum, a researcher studying optimal brain health, discourages television viewing, encourages ambidexterity, and challenges the traditional concept of retirement. Instead, he urges older people to be engaged and productive. Chronic stress accelerates aging, and he emphasizes the role of nutrition, saying that individuals should reduce their caloric intake to 80 percent of what they intend to consume at each meal because overeating and obesity are detrimental to brain health (Nussbaum 2005).

The simplest rule for maintaining brain health is to remember there is a strong correlation between heart health and brain health. Essentially, what is good for the heart is good for the brain. Moreover, people who are obese are at greater risk for diabetes and hypertension. These two conditions increase the risk for cerebrovascular disease, which frequently leads to faulty memory and dementia. The obesity risk of age-related disorders, for example, cardiovascular disease, cancer, and diabetes, is known to be associated with the amount of food ingested. Studies indicate that high food intake increases risk, and low food intake reduces risk. Recent findings suggest that dietary restrictions may enhance resistance of nerve cells in the brain to metabolic damage associated with the development of AD and other neurodegenerative disorders. While further studies are required to establish the extent to which dietary restrictions can lower the incidence of AD, it seems practical to recommend dietary modifications as a preventative approach for age-related disorders, including neurodegenerative disorders (Mattson 2000).

Intellectual and physical activities undertaken by adults between the ages of twenty and sixty seem to offer protection against the development of AD later in life (Friedland et al. 2001). There are also many scientific investigations of elderly individuals who improved their lifestyles by participating in regular exercise and adhering to a healthy diet. Normally, physical exercise increases blood flow, which in turn promotes nerve cell growth. Elders who are attentive to regular health maintenance opportunities, such as getting their immunizations for influenza and pneumonia, controlling their blood pressure, and not smoking, boost their potential to maintain cognitive function in their later years. Some older adults do not fully understand the damaging effects of smoking and few associate smoking with dementia. However, studies have shown that smoking is associated with doubling the risk of dementia and AD (Juan et al. 2004).

Researchers are trying to discover exactly what changes in the brain are responsible for memory and mobility problems. In some cases, imaging helps scientists study brain disorders in living volunteers. The Religious Orders Study consists of hundreds of members of clergy who participate in specific brain research. They all agree to undergo annual, detailed evaluation and eventual brain autopsy. Because many of the changes in the brain that cause AD cannot at this time be examined while a person is alive, participants must agree to brain donation after death. In one such study the data suggested that mild cognitive impairment may be the earliest clinical manifestation of common age-related neurologic diseases (Bennett et al. 2005).

THE THEORY OF COGNITIVE/CEREBRAL RESERVE

The cognitive reserve theory suggests that some people may be better able to withstand the physical attack of AD because they have greater cognitive, or cerebral, reserve. This means that their brains are probably more resilient and able to adapt when subjected to degenerative processes than other individuals. It has also been a helpful analysis when trying to understand individual differences in cognitive aging (Whalley et al. 2004).

Researchers began to ask more questions when, upon autopsy, they found the brains of several nursing home patients had the plaques and tangles that are the disease's signature; yet during their lifetimes these patients displayed no overt symptoms (Stern et al. 2004). The concept of reserve against brain damage stems from the repeated observations that there does not seem to be a direct relationship between the degree of brain pathology and the clinical manifestation of that damage (Stern 2002). There is research that indicates older adults automatically compensate for age-related declines by utilizing brain areas that previously had not played a part in a specific task (Helmuth 1999). Those studied seem to have been able to activate additional brain circuits when other parts of their brains become too damaged by the plaques and tangles to function.

The term *cognitive reserve* has also been used by some researchers when referring to certain physical aspects of the brain, for example, its size and the density of neurons in the outer layer of the brain, known as the cortex. Researchers studied patients who had sustained a traumatic brain injury and learned that a higher level of education and larger brain size before injury may decrease the extent of cognitive deficits following traumatic brain damage (Kesler et al. 2003). Others have defined cognitive reserve as the ability of an individual to compensate for active disease of the brain (Gatz 2005).

Scientific investigations have also concluded that certain health practices can allow some people to cope with the progression of AD better than others, and research suggests these practices may even help prevent AD from developing in the healthy elderly (Scarmeus and Stern 2003). We've covered some of the beneficial habits—good nutrition, smoking cessation, and exercise—but effective stress management and sufficient sleep are important too. Each recommendation for keeping the brain in good working order has value, and older adults are advised to employ as many of the suggestions as possible. Nevertheless, at this time, none are guaranteed to protect all elderly individuals from dementia. For example, there is no convincing evidence that practicing memory exercises and other cognitively stimulating activities are sufficient to prevent AD; it is much more than just a case of "use it or lose it." Since half the people who develop AD are genetically predisposed to the disease, it is important to remember that the results of cognitive training are very specific to the skills that are trained. Also, the types of skills taught by practicing mental puzzles and exercises may be less helpful in everyday life than more commonplace habits such as concentrating, taking notes, or putting objects in the same place each time so that they won't be lost (Gatz 2005).

It is not possible to prevent or cure dementia, although there is extensive research in both areas (Woodward et al. 2005). Nevertheless, researchers are hopeful and older adults are often encouraged to learn new skills. (Take a genealogy class and research your family history, or learn how to use a computer. Line dancing is fun and it is also great exercise.) It was once widely believed that when nerve cells in the adult brain became damaged or died, they were permanently destroyed. But it is now known that the human brain is efficiently and continuously generating new neurons (Kuhn, Palmer, and Fuchs 2001). It is always appropriate to consider ways of reducing the risk of developing dementia with the hope that such approaches may either delay or prevent onset.

The results of current investigations have provided a growing body of evidence that indicates complex mental activities across a life span are associated with a lower risk for dementia and cognitive decline (Caprini et al. 2006; Hall et al. 2006; Valenzuela and Sachdev 2006). A range of life experience that includes educational or occupational accomplishments is increasingly seen as having the potential to provide the brain with the ability to resist impairment due to injury or illness (Stern 2002).

Participation in intellectual and social activities is not only associated with slower cognitive decline in the healthy elderly, but it may also improve well-being and reduce the onset of dementia. Healthcare professionals regularly encourage elderly individuals to keep mentally active by challenging themselves with crossword puzzles, learning new skills, and problem solving. At first glance the advice seems constructive and practical for everyone and certainly benign. However, it is important to keep the recommendations in perspective. It can be risky to accept the perceived benefits of mental exercises as dogma and to assume that if one devotes enough time to challenging intellectual activities one will remain dementia free. This attitude may hold out false hope for some, and those who do develop dementia run the risk of being blamed for their condition, the suspicion being that they did not try hard enough. As an example, when heavy smokers get lung cancer, they are usually viewed as being responsible for their illness and are seen as having contributed to their own fates (Gatz 2005). The decision whether or not to smoke is a matter of choice, but the matter of becoming demented is not.

Still, a focus on preserving cognitive health can improve the quality of life for many older adults. Such efforts may also allow them to continue to actively participate in society, contribute to the economy, and may even help reduce the eventual costs of their care.

CONTROLLING THE DEVELOPMENT OF DEMENTIA: RISK REDUCTION

Although there are certain risk factors that people cannot control, such as genetics and age, there is much that older adults can do to reduce the risks of developing dementia. The three primary areas over which individuals *do* have control are food, activities, and using medications where appropriate.

Increasingly, research consistently shows that lower-fat diets in young and middle-aged adults may reduce the risk for AD decades later. Not all fat is bad, however. Some fats may benefit brain health. One study found that a Mediterranean diet high in olive oil is protective against age-related cognitive decline (Solfrizzi et al. 1999). This might also be true for other unsaturated vegetable oils.

Activities

Physical activity has the ability to improve blood flow to the brain, reduce cardiovascular risk factors, and may also stimulate nerve cell growth and survival. One study of healthy adults between ages sixty and seventy-five revealed mental activities involving planning, scheduling, monitoring, and memory improved in a group participating in aerobic exercise (Small 2002).

Regular exercise to keep hearts healthy has long been recommended by physicians. Along with cardiovascular benefits, new evidence is showing that people who are active during their middle years seem to be at a much lower risk for dementia, particularly AD. Scientists have learned that middle-aged people who exercised at least twice a week had a 50 percent lower chance of developing dementia and a 60 percent lower chance of developing AD than their sedentary peers. The exercise reported was mostly walking and biking strenuously enough to cause sweating and strained breathing.

Another unexpected conclusion of the research was that exercise was found to be most beneficial for those individuals who were predisposed to dementia and AD (Kivipelto et al. 2006). Again, there is evidence that if certain lifestyle habits are identified and treated in middle age, then the prospect of avoiding dementia increases.

Using Medications

As mentioned earlier, high levels of blood cholesterol are a known risk factor for heart disease and there are indications these high levels are also associated with the incidence of AD. Scientists have examined the effect of lowered blood cholesterol on decreasing the risk of developing AD or, at least, reducing the rate of progression. Both population and animal studies have raised the possibility that statins, the most commonly prescribed cholesterol-lowering drugs, may also reduce the risk of dementia. The statin family of medications (lovastatin, pravastatin, simvastatin, and others) are powerful cholesterol-lowering drugs of proven benefit in fighting vascular disease. In one study the risk of developing dementia was found to be reduced by 37 to 50 percent in patients fifty years and older who used statin medicines (Jick et al. 2000).

There are also data confirming that cholesterol has direct effects on the brain, triggering the changes associated with the disease. One key change linked to brain cell death in AD is the buildup of amyloid plaques. Researchers conclude that high levels of cholesterol cause the body to produce more amyloid precursor protein and that effect increases the risk of it being deposited in the brain as amyloid plaques (Koudinov and Koudinova 2001).

Most of the evidence about cholesterol is related to clogged arteries and heart disease. However, scientists have also learned this fatty molecule is an essential component of all cell membranes. Researchers were surprised to find cholesterol may also regulate when and where nerve cells in the brain form the vital junctions known as *synapses*, the structures that help nerve cells communicate with each other (Miller 2001; Travis 2001).

Studies suggesting the possibility of statins blocking or slowing dementia are based primarily on evidence that people with high blood pressure are more likely to develop mild cognitive impairment (MCI). However, a 2005 investigation has found no association between statins and dementia (Zandi et al. 2005). Participants in the study were on average seventy-five years of age. Some speculate statin therapy may need to be started earlier in adulthood or for longer periods to prevent dementia. The point is that (1) it is controversial and (2) *all* drugs have side effects. The use of statins and other lipid-lowering agents by older adults was not associated with a reduced risk of AD or other types of dementia, according to another study of people over sixty-five that appears in *Archives of Neurology* (Rea, Breitner, and Psaty 2005).

As one can tell, the use of statins for the purpose of reducing dementia and AD risk remains controversial. Two clinical studies comparing the occurrence of AD between users and nonusers of statins suggest that risk of AD is substantially reduced among the users. On the other hand, because these studies were not randomized trials, the evidence they produced was insufficient (Scott and Laake 2006).

There are also concerns that statins, which cross the blood-brain barrier, may cause more side effects. The blood-brain barrier is an elaborate meshwork of fine blood vessels and cells, a membrane that acts as a filter allowing certain substances to cross to the brain yet prevents others from crossing. Newer investigations found that adverse events were either infrequently noted or not reported in most of the published studies. As a result, at this time there is insufficient evidence to suggest the use of statins for cognitive improvement in AD patients (Caballero and Nahata 2004). The American Heart Association (AHA) recommends prescribing a dosage no greater than what the patient needs to achieve the goals of therapy. Also, statins need to be selected based on the degree of low-density lipoprotein (LDL) lowering needed and the potential for side effects in each patient.

With the growing recognition of benefits and increased recommendations for cholesterol management, many more patients will require cholesterol-lowering drugs. For most patients, statins are effective for lipid management and have a favorable safety profile.

However, potentially adverse effects have been linked to statin therapy. Cognitive impairment and dementia are two examples that have been reported in some cases. Statins are not benign drugs and all statins share similar adverse effect profiles (King 2003).

Newer research has located a possible link between factors related to cardiovascular disease and AD. One study found that elevated levels of an amino acid called homocysteine, a risk factor for heart disease, are associated with increased risk of developing AD. The relationship between the risk of AD and homocysteine levels is particularly interesting because blood levels of homocysteine can be reduced by increasing intake of folic acid and vitamins B_6 and B_{12}.

A clinical trial funded by the National Institute on Aging is currently studying whether reducing homocysteine levels with folic acid and vitamin B_6 and B_{12} supplements will slow the rate of cognitive decline in older adults with AD (NIA 2006).

Other investigation on risk factors for dementia including AD has focused on studying the physical and psychological impact that stress in early life has on the adult brain. Early life stress (ELS) has been found to affect the shape of areas of the brain, and this may reflect the influence of traumatic events (Cohen 2006). In another study, ELS has been associated with a range of adverse outcomes in adults including abnormalities in electrical brain activity and personality and increased susceptibility to substance abuse and depression (McFarlane 2005).

Memory loss and impaired cognitive abilities brought about by such stresses as neglect and abuse during infancy may be triggered by a hormone produced in the brain. It was once thought that high levels of steroid stress hormones produced by the body's adrenal glands were responsible. A new study found that the corticotropin-releasing hormone (CRH) may be responsible for cell death in the area of the brain that controls memory. If further research can find a way to block the actions of CRH on the brain, then it will be possible to develop new, more effective ways to prevent late-life cognitive impairment (Brunson et al. 2001).

MEMORY: HOW IT WORKS AND
HOW IT IS AFFECTED BY AGING

Memory is the process by which information and experiences can be acquired, stored, and eventually recalled. Although it frequently takes longer for adults over age fifty to learn new information, once it is understood, the material is as well remembered by an older adult as by someone younger. Most mature individuals, particularly those over age sixty-five, admit to having some problems with remembering. They may even convince themselves that they are developing a dementia such as AD. However, the statistics show that only about 3 percent of people between sixty-five and seventy-four actually have AD (Griffin 2005).

Memory loss is also one of the major worries of the baby boomers. They are watching their parents suffer with AD or other dementias and speculate about their own potential vulnerability to such illnesses. A 2006 study on memory disclosed that although well-educated older participants worried their mental abilities were weakening, they took a practical and effective approach: they used their apprehension as an incentive to actively practice physical and mental exercises in order to prevent these deficits from materializing (Dark-Freudeman, West, and Viverito 2006).

Serious memory problems are those that affect a person's ability to successfully complete everyday activities. Shopping and handling money are typical examples of standard tasks all adults generally accomplish effectively. However, when an individual gets lost in formerly familiar places or is not able to follow directions and asks repetitive questions, it generally indicates a serious memory problem.

Memory is an extraordinarily complex function that is made up of diverse components and processes. Each type of memory is joined to a particular kind of brain function. As an example, long-term memory, the kind people are most familiar with, is used to store facts, observations, and life histories. Working (or short-term) memory is used to hold the same kind of information but for a much shorter amount of time, often just long enough for it to be useful.

Human memory is an abstract relationship among thoughts that arises out of neural activity spread over the whole brain. When someone experiences an event, the brain uses everything in the environment—sights, smells, sounds, and personal impressions—to develop an association or link with the event for retrieval at a later time. That connection is the memory of the event. People remember something best if learned in a context they understand, particularly if it has an emotional impact (Ranpura 2000).

Handling information to be remembered is done in steps: acquiring, retaining, and recalling facts. Information comes from the outside world into the centers in the brain, which register whatever the five senses perceive. However, very few people are consciously aware of everything going on around them, and awareness occurs only if they are trained to deliberately focus their attention in that manner. When that happens, the impressions of the environment or of a situation are placed in short-term memory.

Psychologists refer to small amounts of related information as a "chunk." A chunk refers to digits, words, chess positions, or people's faces, for example. The ability of the brain to recognize chunks affects the capacity of short-term memory. The popular theory that short-term memory could hold only five to nine chunks (seven, plus or minus two) has been widely accepted by researchers for many years (Miller 1956). These concepts are basic elements of all subsequent theories of memory.

Understand that the capacity of working memory is limited. In fact, newer research suggests that a person can concentrate on about only four items at one time. Therefore, individuals must take one of the following actions with regard to each piece of information that comes into this short-term storage area: (1) continuously rehearse it, so that it stays there; (2) move it out of this area by shifting it to long-term memory; or (3) move it out of this area by forgetting it (Cowan 2001).

FORGETTING

Forgetting (sometimes referred to by researchers as *retention loss*) can be either a spontaneous or a gradual process in which a person is unable to recall old memories from specific memory-storing areas of the brain. Most people seem to notice only the few things they have forgotten and overlook the enormous amount of information they have remembered. Still, this does not diminish the frustration individuals experience when they are unable to recall a name or an object in a timely manner.

The effectiveness of working memory is closely linked to a person's ability to effectively prioritize what is important. A common example is of someone driving on a highway with squabbling children in the backseat. The careful driver will ignore the less important information (the bickering children) in favor of the more important, namely, driving safely (Blasko 2005).

Some researchers propose that people who have better focusing abilities are more skilled when initially processing information. They suggest that if something is forgotten, it is because the individual either never really learned the information in the first place (failure to focus) or learned it for a brief period of time then forgot it (Blasko 2005).

Although an individual's brain registers all data the senses acquire, it retains only information deemed meaningful. If information is not used or reinforced, it may simply fade away. The most frequent reason for forgetting information is difficulty in transferring it from working memory to long-term memory. In addition, people may "forget" because of an inability to recall information stored in long-term memory (Vockell 2006).

Long-term memory has an unlimited capacity to retain information, yet data retrieval is not always reliable. For example, everyone has had the experience in which we *know* we know something, but it slips our mind. This irritating event is referred to as *tip-of-the-tongue phenomenon* (TOT). TOT has intrigued psychologists for nearly a century. Brown and McNeil (1966) provided the first systematic exploration of the phenomenon, and findings since their significant study suggest the following:

- TOTs are a nearly universal experience.
- They occur about once a week.
- People notice an increase in TOTs as they grow older.
- A common example is the inability to recall a proper name.
- They are resolved during the experience about half the time.

Forgetting as a result of AD occurs because of damage sustained by the hippocampus, a brain structure essential for the formation of both short-term and long-term memories (ADEAR 2006). If the hippocampus is gradually being destroyed, the patient cannot form new memories. Also, although memory formation occurs in the hippocampus, memories are probably not stored there exclusively.

THE TRUTH ABOUT BRAIN BOOSTERS

People who sell unproven health remedies have been around for ages. Today, there are more outlets for quacks to peddle their wares to hopeful, often desperate clients. In addition to TV, radio, magazines, newspapers, infomercials, mail, and even word-of-mouth, there is the global marketplace of the Internet. Countless Web sites advertise rapid healing and offer miracle cures. Typically, older adults are targeted for such scams. In fact, a government study has found the majority of victims of healthcare scams are over age sixty-five.

Many people worry about their memories fading and growing less dependable as they age. Consequently, they are easily lured by the appeal of tempting but unproven remedies. Two examples are so-called smart pills that promise to strengthen cognition and removal of amalgam dental fillings because of their suggested toxicity. And for all the legitimate brain-retraining exercises that help, there are many more that are worthless (NIA 2002). Many brain-retraining exercises are limited in their effectiveness, and it is unclear how or if regular brain workouts are able to postpone AD. More research is needed. Nevertheless, exercising the brain has long been encouraged (crossword puzzles, learning new skills, and so on). They are not *universally* effective because of so many variables—elders with advanced disease, other sensory impairments, unspecified physical or mental health issues—but they still have value.

There are several FDA-approved medications that may help clarify thinking and augment memory and alertness in people with AD and certain other cognitive impairments. These "smart pills" are also known as nootropic drugs, for example, cognitive enhancers made up of chemicals that have a mild to moderate effect on improving some individuals' problems with memory and cognition; donepezil, galantamine, and rivastigmine are examples of drugs prescribed for patients with AD. Modanifil is prescribed to improve alertness and also to relieve conditions such as narcolepsy and the fatigue accompanying fibromyalgia and chronic fatigue syndrome. (And it may still be used by college students cramming for exams.) Many claim it helps their memories, so some physicians prescribed it off-label to help AD patients who display apathy. Some patients use it along with antidepressants to manage depression that featured apathy.

The concept and definition of a nootropic drug was first proposed in 1972 by a Belgian scientist, C. E. Giurgea. He devised the term *nootropic* to describe a classification of drugs that enhance learning and memory (Giurgea 1973).

The public needs to remain skeptical when evaluating extravagant claims for mental improvement. A broad array of compounds, including certain vitamins, herbs, and medications that are reputed to improve such mental functions as memory and alertness or to lessen or prevent damage to brain cells, can be referred to as "smart pills."

Another quackery involves teeth fillings. Amalgam dental fillings are the common silver variety, which are made up of an amalgam of silver, tin, and mercury. Roughly 50 percent of the mix is mercury, and that combination is where the problem lies. Mercury is toxic and the two routes known to be most hazardous in humans are (1) direct contact with the skin and (2) breathing in mercury vapors. During dental procedures a small amount of mercury vapor is released throughout the installation or removal of silver fillings. In laboratory conditions mercury has been shown to affect nerve cells and some of the biochemical processes involved in AD. No evidence exists, however, to show any connection between mercury-based fillings and AD or any other neurological diseases. The FDA, the US Public Health Service, and the World Health Organization continue to support the use of amalgam for dental treatments (Saxe et al. 1999; Clarkson 2003).

Enthusiastic, anecdotal testimony of unproven remedies encourages false hope and may even be physically harmful to a patient. Furthermore, fraudulent claims can cause unnecessary expenses and often deter people from getting necessary medical treatment. One reason these scams flourish is that they target people who are worried, anxious, and sometimes desperate. It can be very tempting to accept without question the false promise of a quick, guaranteed cure.

People need to be vigilant in protecting themselves from health scams. Consequently, the public is urged to question what they see and read in ads or on the Internet and to look for red flags in ads or promotional material that

- Promises a quick or painless cure
- Claims to be made from a special, secret, or ancient formula—often only available by mail or from one sponsor
- Uses testimonials or undocumented case histories from satisfied patients
- Claims to be effective for a wide range of ailments
- Claims to cure a disease that is not yet fully understood by medical science, such as arthritis or cancer
- Offers an additional "free" gift or a larger amount of the product as a "special promotion"
- Requires advance payment and claims limited availability of the product (NIA 2002)

If you have questions about a product, talk to your doctor or contact one of the following organizations. Always get the facts about health products and protect yourself from scams.

- Quackwatch, Inc., is a nonprofit corporation making information available to combat health-related frauds, myths, fads, and fallacies. Go to http://www.quackwatch.org.
- US Postal Inspection Service Office of Investigation. Check the phone book for the number of your local postal inspector or go to http://www.usps.com/postalinspectors/fraud.
- Write to the Council of Better Business Bureaus:

> Council of Better Business Bureaus (CBBB)
> 1200 Wilson Boulevard
> 8th Floor
> Arlington, VA 22203

Check the phone book for the number of your local chapter, or go to http://www.bbb.org.

Contact the US Food and Drug Administration at:

> FDA
> 5600 Fishers Lane
> Rockville, MD 20857-0001
> Phone: 1-888-INFO-FDA
> (1-888-463-6332 toll free)
> www.fda.gov

PROTECTING AND STRENGTHENING COGNITIVE PERFORMANCE

At this time there is no uniform definition of what constitutes cognitive health. Researchers are still struggling to create a comprehensive definition. Clearly, cognitive health includes the absence of cognitive decline, but the term goes well beyond that and should take into account optimal mental functioning. A 2001 workshop titled The Healthy Brain, conducted by the National Institutes of Health, concluded that cognition "should not be defined simply as the absence of diseases such as Alzheimer's disease. While the study of cognitive health cannot ignore dementia, the definition of cognitive health has many different aspects and should emphasize successful aging instead of normal aging." The concept of successful aging embraces the more positive aspects of aging, whereas normal aging is frequently used to describe declines associated with the aging process.

Research has shown there are both physical and mental factors that seem to influence which older adults can retain their intellectual function. In the absence of organic disease, the brain that is challenged and stimulated regularly will function longer and better than the inactive brain.

Newer investigations emphasize the importance of years of education as a safeguard from age-related cognitive decline. Brain imaging showed increased frontal lobe activity in well-educated older adults when they were taking memory tests. This finding was the opposite of what happened in younger adults during a similar test. The research suggested that more years of education strengthens an individual's ability to develop alternative networks in the brain. Furthermore, highly educated people are known to remain more active physically and mentally as they age, which also has a beneficial effect on cognition (Stern et al. 2002; Springer et al. 2005).

Education, with its attendant reading, studying, and testing, appears to increase the number and strength of synaptic connections. The more connections or synapses one has between brain cells, the more resistant they are to the effects of AD and other dementias (Kotulak 1997). Vigorous physical activity improves blood flow to the brain and optimizes lung function, which, in turn, ensures that the blood is adequately oxygenated. Another important aspect of intact cognition is the importance of remaining socially engaged. Individuals who curtail their social activities are at risk for cognitive decline (Mitka 2001; NIH 2001).

A reexamination of available research has begun to focus public health scrutiny on lifestyle changes to help maintain cognitive performance. Although much more research is needed in this area, the good news is that many of these approaches, such as controlling weight and blood pressure, staying physically active, and being involved in the community, are the same behaviors that many people have already adopted for their physical and emotional health.

OPTIMIZING COGNITIVE SKILLS: EXERCISES TO RETRAIN THE BRAIN

A number of studies have demonstrated that it is possible to improve performance in such cognitive skills as face-name memory and problem-solving tasks (Willis 1990). Many researchers believe that the brain has numerous untapped pathways. Their theory is that by stimulating those pathways in new ways, it is possible to increase the number and size of the brain's synaptic connections—its key electrical circuits. They also believe that the growth of new brain cells contributes to cognitive reserve. Neurons are the fundamental building blocks of the cerebral cortex and serve as the brain's primary network communicators. For decades, it was believed that the neurons communicated only with one another. However, recent research has discovered that some glial cells* may also contribute to cortical communications. Neurons operate the sensory systems necessary for data

---

*Glial (Greek for glue) cells help neurons remain in their appropriate places in the cerebral cortex.

intake, the decision-making systems in the frontal lobes dedicated to informational processing, and the motor systems that carry out our decisions by executing the actions we take or the movements we make.

While all researchers agree that aging affects everyone's mental abilities to some extent, the range of differences is very broad. Current investigations indicate there are many older adults who are using alternative brain networks to compensate for circuits that have lost their function. This strongly suggests that the elaborate networks and structures inside the brain go through modification, reorganization, and cellular adjustment. The changes are reflected in substantial transformations in the brain (Stern 2002). Meanwhile, those individuals with low cognitive reserve do not have this ability.

The Seattle Longitudinal Study, initiated by K. Warner Schaie, involved more than five thousand people, ages twenty to over ninety. The purpose of the study was to determine what happens to the intellectual abilities of aging people. It was concluded that intellectual decline varies widely and depends largely on intellectual stimulation (Schaie 2005).

Several factors stood out in the findings regarding elders who maintain their mental acumen. Among them are:

- A high standard of living reflective of an above-average education and income
- Absence of chronic diseases
- A commitment to reading, travel, cultural events, and professional associations

Cognitive exercises in old age can boost intellectual power, help maintain mental functions like problem solving, and may help to reverse memory decline. Even if an older adult has not had the advantage of a good early education, there is still much that can be done to enhance intellectual ability.

Just as physical activity keeps the body strong, mental activity keeps the mind alert and responsive. Ongoing learning stimulates the brain's ability to grow and adapt because when the brain is active, it produces new dendrites, the connections between nerve cells that allow cells to communicate with one another. This helps the brain store and retrieve information more easily.

Examples of mental activities that can help to improve cognitive functioning include:

- Reading; join a book club and exchange ideas with others
- Doing something artistic
- Taking a course
- Playing games—puzzles, crosswords, chess, and other board games are all great for sparking brain activity
- Learning about technology—there are always new things to learn about computers and new ways to use them. (Do you use a mouse with your computer? Train yourself to use the touchpad.)
- Learning to play a musical instrument (OASIS 2004)

CAN FOOD AFFECT MEMORY?

Food as a component of good health is so basic that it is frequently taken for granted. Keeping a nourishing diet is an essential life habit that generally can protect health and delay disability. Yet good nutrition and a healthy diet may well be the most overlooked areas for healthy aging since clinicians often fail to screen their elderly patients for nutritional risk (CDC 2006; English 2006).

Only recently has a concerted effort been made to understand the mechanisms by which food may alter memory. A promising area of research focused on highly active molecules called *free radicals*. As we age, damage from these free radicals can accumulate in nerve cells and result in a loss of cell function that may contribute to AD (Morley 2001).

Free radicals are highly reactive atoms in molecules that can potentially injure cells and may be responsible for numerous age-related diseases.

If free radicals are not neutralized by antioxidants, they have the capability of damaging cells, blood vessels, and organs through a process called *oxidative stress*. Oxidative stress is an important cause of brain degeneration. A number of studies suggested that antioxidants from dietary supplements or food might provide some protection from the harm caused by oxidative stress (NIH 2006). Although it is doubtful that the cure for AD lies within nutritional guidelines, it may at least delay its onset.

The findings from several research reports strongly suggest that concentrations of homocysteine, an amino acid found in the blood, is related not only to a higher risk of coronary heart disease, stroke, and peripheral vascular disease, but also to lower cognitive function in older adults (Elias et al. 2005).

Most people with a high homocysteine level do not get enough folic acid, vitamin B_6, or vitamin B_{12} in their diet. However, insufficient vitamin B_{12} generally causes confusion and disorientation, symptoms that simulate dementia.

These are essential vitamins that can help homocysteine return to normal levels. Other possible causes of homocysteine elevations include low levels of thyroid hormone, kidney disease, psoriasis, and certain medications (AAFP 2006).

Recent investigation of elevated homocysteine levels and mental function found that although vitamin treatment did lower homocysteine levels, cognition did not improve (Clarke 2006; McMahon et al. 2006).

Nonetheless, diet-related factors do play an important role in the cognitive functioning of older adults. There is evidence to show that diet can have an effect on cognitive impairment and cognitive decline in older age particularly through its impact on vascular diseases. There is a significant relationship between mental processes and the intake of various nutrients, such as polyunsaturated fatty acids, antioxidant vitamins, folic acid, and vitamin B_{12} (Andel 2005).

The brain is one of several organs susceptible to damage caused by oxidative stress. Furthermore, there is increasing evidence that oxidative stress is involved in cerebral aging and dementia. After carefully analyzing earlier studies, investigators have found that research has consistently proposed that diet-related factors play an important role in cognitive functions in aging (Deschamps et al. 2001).

However, the concept of how cognition can be affected by a person's eating habits is controversial. Research has shown that saturated fat and cholesterol intake increases the risk of cardiovascular disease and that cardiovascular disease is linked to dementia. Significantly, vascular dementia is most strongly related to saturated fat intake. Of particular interest is the fact that fish consumption, which is associated with a high intake of omega-3 fatty acids, is inversely related to dementia (Kalmijn et al. 1997). The conclusion was that increasing fish consumption might reduce the incidence of dementia.

Recently the results of a significant study reported in the *Archives of Neurology* strongly recommended eating fish three times a week in order to reduce an individual's risk of incurring AD and other dementias. Scientists studied nine hundred elderly men and women and learned that the participants with the highest levels of the omega-3 fatty acid DHA at the beginning of the study were 47 percent less likely to develop dementia and 39 percent less likely to get AD during the investigation than the rest of the group. These conclusions were reached after the participants, who had mental skills tests every two years, were followed on average for nine years (Morris 2006; Schaefer 2006).

As a practical matter the American Heart Association realizes that most Americans are not going to eat the oily, fatty fish that is the source of the valuable omega-3 fatty acids three times a week, so AHA recommend using supplements.

Remember: what is good for the heart is good for the brain.

DHA (docosahexaenoic acid) and EPA (eicosapentaenoic) are omega-3 fatty acids belonging to the class of nutrients called essential fatty acids. They are found in salmon, sardines, lake trout, mackerel, and herring and play an important role in dementia risk reduction.

Source: American Heart Association, "Diet and Lifestyle Recommendations 2006"

Generally, elderly individuals are recognized as the largest group in society at greatest risk for nutritional deficiency (ADA 2000). Research shows that cognitive decline and dementia are associated with lifestyle and vascular factors. However, there are still unanswered questions about the specific role of dietary fats in developing mental impairments.

Scientists have known for some time that cognitive decline is linked to diabetes and more specifically because of the effect glucose seems to have on memory. When glucose concentrations in patients with dementia of the AD type were increased, their cognition improved (Craft et al. 1996). This improvement appears to be dependent on the increase in insulin concentrations made by elevated glucose concentrations. The early results are further supported by studies showing that poor glucose control in diabetics is generally associated with impaired cognition (Morley 2000). The investigations demonstrate that when the glucose concentration returns to normal, cognition improves. Hyperglycemia per se can have a harmful effect on cognition. Furthermore, when patients with long-term, poorly controlled diabetes develop small infarcts, the destruction of tissue due to impaired blood supply in the central nervous system can result in vascular dementia that produces permanent memory dysfunction.

Researchers have known for decades that even modest deficits in nutrition can cause alterations in the mental status of older adults (Goodwin, Goodwin, and Garry 1983). In addition, elders are at risk for developing anorexia and malnutrition because as a group they have more illnesses and take more medications. Both conditions are very common in elderly individuals (Morley 1997).

At the Tenth International Conference on Alzheimer's Disease and Related Disorders (ICAD), sponsored by the Alzheimer's Association, additional information was presented that strongly supported previous findings regarding the influence of nutrition on mental function (Hitti 2006). The research determined that a high intake of saturated fat from milk products at mid-life was associated with poorer overall mental status and memory, and the risk of mild cognitive impairment more than doubled. On the other hand, a high intake of polyunsaturated fatty acids was associated with better memory, as was frequent fish consumption, which was also linked to better mental/physical coordination, reasoning, and decision making (Laitinen et al. 2004).

The part dietary supplements play in reducing widespread, age-related health issues is still unclear. However, there is an area of discussion in which all healthcare professionals are in agreement. They are unified in pointing out that lifestyle modifications, including dietary modification and regular exercise, have the potential to diminish the incidence of the cognitive age-related diseases.

> For more information about dietary supplements, visit http://ods.od.nih.gov.

Adequate nutrition is essential for healthy aging, the prevention or delay of chronic diseases and disease-related disabilities, the treatment and management of chronic diseases, and an individual's overall quality of life. The Administration on Aging (AoA) directs the Elderly Nutrition Program, a nation-wide plan that provides grants to support nutrition services for older people throughout the country. The legislative intent is to make community-based food services available to older adults who may be at risk of losing their independence. Examples of services are the hot lunches regularly served in senior centers, some churches, and various other settings for elders who have problems meeting their nutritional needs. The reasons range from no longer being able to drive and personal economic shortfalls to social isolation and the inability to prepare cooked meals. Meals-on-Wheels is another essential nutrition service for homebound elders. Those are the risks these elders face and the Elderly Nutrition Program fills a critical need.

The nutrition services observe ethnic and religious traditions and offer many social opportunities for elders to create informal support networks, thus forming new friendships and fulfilling social needs. An additional benefit is that most community meal sites also make available a wide variety of health and wellness resources for participants.

Chapter 7
Falls
Accidents That Will Happen

Dementia is a widespread, inherent, and sometimes deadly cause of falls. Falls occur frequently in the cognitively impaired, and sometimes even the most conscientious of caregivers may not be able to prevent them. Nevertheless, it is important to understand why they happen and what can be done to reduce both the occurrence and the consequences.

A fall in old age can be a life-altering event, a fact to which the thousands of elderly persons who fall each year can attest. In addition to the obvious and readily correctible fall hazards—loose scatter rugs, trailing wires from electrical outlets, or insufficient lighting—older adults are potentially easy victims of the many random threats to their safety and well-being. This occurs because the whole process of aging inevitably brings about alterations in physical, emotional, and cognitive abilities.

The cause of falls ranges from the complex, such as the neurodegenerative changes in the brain that can affect an individual's gait and ability to assess obstacles, to something as simple as having a piece of furniture out of place. Caregivers want to keep their loved ones safe while allowing them to enjoy as much independence as possible without unduly restricting their movements.

It has long been known that the annual incidence of falls for patients with dementia is twice that of the cognitively normal population (Tinetti, Speechly, and Ginter 1988). It is estimated that about half of the falls in this group result in injuries and, significantly, many end in hip fractures and increased mortality.

FALL RISKS

While all age groups are susceptible, 60 percent of fall-related deaths occur among people sixty-five and older. Each year, more than one-third of the elderly in the United States falls (Tinetti 2003). Falls are the number-one cause of injury-related death for males age eighty and older and for females age seventy-five and older. Furthermore, should a fall victim sustain a hip fracture, the increase in mortality is significant. Twenty-five percent of those who do sustain a hip fracture die within one year, and another 50 percent never return to their prior level of mobility or independence (Jackson 2002).

Most falls are due to multiple factors and need to be investigated for more than one cause. Typically, the risks for falls are classified as intrinsic or extrinsic. Intrinsic risks are age-related changes that can impair systems involved in maintaining balance and stability (for example, while standing, walking, or sitting). Extrinsic hazards arise from environmental factors that can increase the risk of falls independently or when they act together with intrinsic factors (Merck 2005).

A recent study in the *American Journal of Public Health* examined fall rates of adults forty-five and older. The researchers determined that middle-aged and older adults are at higher risk for falling outdoors rather than indoors. Most of these occurred while walking outdoors, where the environment was largely composed of uneven surfaces and curbs. Participants who were frail and in questionable health were at a greater risk for indoor falls (Li et al. 2005).

Figure 7.1. Examples of Intrinsic and Extrinsic Fall Risks

Intrinsic	Extrinsic
Age	Unfamiliar surroundings (for example, relocating to a new home)
Previous fall	Polypharmacy, alcohol
Vertigo	Clutter
Gait disorder, deconditioning	Absence of grab bars in bathroom, nonskid mats in tub, shower
Sensory deficits, such as in vision and hearing	Improper footwear, slippery floors, poor lighting
Medical conditions, for example, dementia, stroke, macular degeneration, incontinence	Unsafe stairways, uneven floors

Virginia, seventy-two and recently diagnosed with AD, lives at home with her seventy-eight-year-old husband, Frank. As the primary caregiver, Frank managed fairly well balancing his part-time supermarket job and taking care of his wife. Virginia had been alone for the few hours Frank was away working, and since there never had been a problem before, he saw no reason to change the routine. However, he came home one afternoon and found her on the floor, with her right leg at an odd angle. Apparently when she attempted to put a leash on their dog she tripped over the leash and fell on a small end table.

Virginia's fall caused a hip fracture that resulted not only in surgery and a lengthy rehabilitation, but also a marked deterioration in her quality of life and a questionable prognosis.

Every fall is a potential crisis for an individual with dementia. Those with mild to moderate dementia are potentially very vulnerable, and, when they sustain a fall, it is often followed by devastating consequences. Regardless of the cause, the aftermath of a fall can be ruinous and it often irreparably alters the lives of patients and their families.

Statistics show that every hour an older adult dies as the result of a fall. In 2001 more than eleven thousand people over sixty-five died as a result of a fall. Among the elderly, 54 percent of fatal falls occurred in the home. Most falls happen to women, in their homes, in the afternoon (NIAMS 2005). Falls are also the leading cause of severe nonfatal injuries, and they are a frequent cause of hospital admissions (CDC 2002).

Healthcare professionals have long known that fractures in older adults may contribute to the risk of early death (Alexander 1999; Sterling, O'Connor, and Bonadies 2001). A sizeable percentage of hip fracture patients die within a year of their injury (Leibson et al. 2002). Virginia was in that percentage. Although she survived her surgery, her therapeutic rehabilitation was unsuccessful. She subsequently developed a foot drop, never regained her ability to walk, and died within a few months of her fall.

Deaths from chronic diseases have declined because they are managed so much more effectively than in times past. However, the geriatric death rate caused by falling has risen sharply since the 1990s (AP 2006). Most fractures among older adults are caused by falls (Bell, Talbot-Stern, and Hennessy 2000) and nearly a third of the people who do fall suffer severe injuries such as head traumas and hip fractures. Inevitably, these episodes become the leading causes of fatalities (Leibson et al. 2002).

FALL PREVENTION: MEDICAL MANAGEMENT, PHYSICAL ACTIVITY, AND ENVIRONMENTAL MODIFICATION

Falls in the elderly population have many different causes. Accordingly, researchers have confirmed that the most effective fall-prevention programs have several components. First, in order to successfully reduce fall risks, an individual needs to recognize the hazards. Professionals can then help to identify risks and develop a plan that involves both patients and families. Specific physical activities can be aimed at reducing falls by increasing balance and mobility skills. How does the individual go up and down stairs or get in and out of a chair or car? Does she need a cane, a walker, or a wheelchair? How far is she able to walk? When walking, is her gait abnormal? Does she limp, drag her feet, or stagger? These are some common questions to consider.

Physical therapists develop exercises to remedy weaknesses. Occupational therapists may suggest splints to support joints and recommend helpful devices that include a bath stool in the shower or tub; grab bars around the toilet or tub; and long-handled shoehorns and sock grippers. In addition, certain changes can be tailored to the home and community environment that will reduce hazards and allow elderly individuals to complete their daily activities in relative safety.

Medical Management

Initially, it is important to talk with a health professional about getting a risk assessment for falling. This can be done during a routine visit to a primary care physician. Some of the more common health factors that can contribute to fall injuries are taking multiple medications, osteoporosis, being over age eighty, changes in balance and walking patterns, and deficits in vision and hearing.

Physical Activity

Physical activity is beneficial for the health of people of all ages, including the older population. It can reduce the likelihood of certain chronic diseases, may relieve symptoms of depression, helps to maintain independent living, and enhances overall quality of life (SG 2004). Research has shown that even in late life, mobility and functioning can be improved through physical activity. Studies also show that balance, flexibility, and strength training not only improve mobility but also help reduce the chance of falling (Butler et al. 1998).

There are many creative, low-impact forms of physical fitness and strength training that can greatly improve an older adult's ability to avoid falls or to boost recovery outcomes in case of an accident. Few seniors exercise regularly and, consequently, this lack of conditioning makes it more difficult to recover from a fall.

Environmental Modification

The environment in which elderly people live presents a wide variety of potential dangers. At home older adults need to be concerned about slips, trips, and falls. Safety can be improved by making some practical changes. Older people tend to live in older homes that often need repairs and modernizing. Over 60 percent of older adults live in homes that are more than twenty years old. Suitable home modification and repair can accommodate physical and lifestyle changes, thereby increasing comfort and security. For example, the bathroom can be modified by installing grab bars in the shower or tub, providing something to sit on, and having nonslip surfaces. Water temperatures can be lowered to 120°F to prevent scalding. Stairs need to have handrails and adequate lighting.

Loss of footing also results from using household objects that were intended for other purposes, for example, climbing on kitchen chairs or balancing on boxes or books to increase height. (For more on home safety, see figure 7.2.)

There are many trip and fall hazards in the community, such as uneven or cracked sidewalks, tree roots, and potholes. Trying to cross the street in some neighborhoods can be dangerous if there are no traffic lights or vehicle speed is excessive.

Normal aging markedly affects vision by reducing contrast sensitivity, depth perception, and color vision, important factors to consider when older adults participate in both indoor and outdoor activities. A senior who generally has good visual acuity may still have difficulty seeing outdoors on bright sunny days, cloudy days, or if outdoor areas are poorly lit. For patients with dementia, the environment is a critical factor for their well-being. Families and caregivers need to recognize potential hazards in the home and take the steps to correct them. Falls are the leading cause of injury-related death and the most common cause of nonfatal injuries and hospital admissions for trauma among people sixty-five and older. In 2000, 1.6 million seniors were seen in emergency departments for fall injuries, and 353,000 were hospitalized (CDC 2001).

Figure 7.2. Home Safety: Problems and Solutions

Typical problem	Suggested solution
Difficulty getting in and out off the shower	Install grab bars, shower seals, or transfer benches
Slipping in the tub or shower	Place nonskid strips or decals in tub and shower
Difficulty in turning faucet handles/doorknobs	Replace with lever handles
Access to home	Install ramps; if accessibility problem is temporary, it is often possible to rent a ramp
Inadequate heating or ventilation	Install insulation, storm windows, and air conditioning
Difficulty climbing stairs	Install bilateral handrails for support; install or rent chair lift system

---

CDC Resources

To learn more about environmental modification strategies for fall prevention, look for the National Center for Injury Prevention and Control on the Internet at http://www.cdc.gov/ncipc or contact by phone at 770-488-1506. The following brochures are available free of charge and provide an overview of home safety measures to prevent falls in older adults. They are also available in Spanish or Chinese.

- Check for Safety: A Home Fall-Prevention Checklist for Older Adults (099-6156)
- Check for Safety (099-6590)
- What YOU Can Do to Prevent Falls (099-6589)

DECONDITIONING AND HIP FRACTURES

Families responsible for someone with dementia can increase the safety level of their caregiving when they know the risks and know how to modify or eliminate them.

Approximately three hundred thousand older adults suffer fall-related hip fractures each year (CDC 2002). Although hip fracture victims are overwhelmingly female, the fracture rate in both sexes increases exponentially with age (Samelson, Zhang, and Kiel 2002).

The typical hip fracture patient profile is that of an elderly woman with dementia who sustains a fall and may or may not complain of severe hip pain, but she is unable to walk (Brunner, Eshilian-Oates, and Kuo 2003). Cognitive impairment is a key warning sign for hip fracture risk. Other red flags are ministrokes, or transient ischemic attacks (TIAs), and previous fractures (Marcantonio et al. 2001).

Hospital stays are almost twice as long for elderly patients who are admitted after a fall than for other reasons (Dunn et al. 1992). Excessive bed rest is a common and hazardous feature of their hospitalization. Deconditioning soon develops because being confined to bed causes at least a 10 percent loss of leg muscle strength in one week. The deconditioning also affects both cardiac and respiratory systems, which subsequently undermines an individual's capacity for optimal exercising. Trying to reverse the situation is not only very difficult but it can also be a tedious, protracted effort (Hoeing and Rubenstein 1991).

Geriatric patients hospitalized for hip fracture surgery face the possibility of many postoperative complications. However, they also must become mobile as soon as possible after surgery in order to improve their overall functioning. Delays in getting these patients out of bed after surgery are associated with both poor functioning and survival. Furthermore, it is important to note that one-fifth of patients with hip fractures are admitted to the hospital with major clinical abnormalities such as heart failure, serious electrolyte imbalance, or respiratory failure. If a patient has even more than *one* abnormality before having surgery, the risk of postoperative problems increases almost tenfold (McLaughlin et al. 2006).

On average, many geriatric hip fracture patients are immobilized approximately five days during their hospital stay. A longer period of immobilization is associated with a poor functional outcome. This requires serious consideration because it can make the difference between being able to go home or not. Furthermore, prolonged immobilization is also linked to increased mortality (Siu et al. 2006).

Compared with individuals who do not fall, elderly fall victims will experience a greater inability to regain skill and confidence in resuming their activities of daily living (ADLs). Falls affect virtually all physical and social activities (Kiel, O'Sullivan, and Teno 1991). Consequently, these developments soon place them at a far greater risk for later institutionalization (Tinetti, Lui, and Claus 1993).

FALL DYNAMICS AND DEFENSES

Let's discuss the three elements that play essential roles in fractures due to falls, which make up the fracture triangle:

(1) *The fall.* Essentially, a fall is the result of losing one's footing or traction, for example, as when walking on a wet or slippery surface. Aging contributes to falls because it brings about diminished reaction time and delayed reflexes. Moreover, inadequate reaction time makes it harder to regain balance following a sudden movement or shift of body weight.

(2) *The force and direction of the fall.* The force of a fall determines whether the individual will sustain a fracture. For example, the greater the distance of the hip bone to the ground, the greater the chance of incurring a hip fracture. Consequently, being tall increases one's risk of a hip fracture. The path of the fall is also an important consideration: falling sideways or straight down is more risky than falling backward. Trying to break a fall with one's hands or by grabbing onto something mid-fall will help prevent the fracture (NIAMS 2005).

Initial investigations have suggested that by wearing trochanteric (hip) padding, people can decrease the chances of fracturing a hip after a fall. The protective device is made up with plastic shields or foam pads that fit into the pockets of specially designed underwear. The hip pad acts as a shock absorber, distributing the fall's energy throughout the pad, thereby lessening the impact to the hip.

Hip protectors may be effective in reducing damage following a fall for elderly nursing home residents with a previous history of hip fracture. The devices are particularly appealing because they offer a noninvasive, nonpharmaceutical solution to a grave health problem.

There is no evidence, however, that hip protectors are effective in reducing the incidence of hip fracture following a fall among elders living in the community. In one study, general complaints reported were discomfort, skin irritation, and abrasions, which led to a general lack of compliance (Thorpe 2004).

(3) **Bone fragility.** The most prevalent cause of falls in the elderly, primarily women, results from *osteoporosis*, popularly called the brittle bone disease, a significant decrease in bone density. An estimated 10 million Americans over fifty have osteoporosis. Another 46 million have a related condition, also characterized by low bone mass, that is called *osteopenia* (FORE 2007). However, in osteopenia the bone loss is not as severe. Osteoporosis is by far the more serious disorder, but osteopenia is a precursor for developing osteoporosis.

People lose bone mass very slowly over a long period of time. Adults reach peak bone mass at about age thirty, but bones change constantly throughout life by means of a process known as *remodeling*. This process involves two major types of bone cells: *osteoclasts*, which break down old or worn bone, thereby creating bone cavities, and *osteoblasts*, which fill in the cavities. If the amount of new bone equals the amount being dissolved, bones stay strong. However, several factors can cause the balance to shift so that bones become weaker and more brittle, thus putting affected individuals at high risk for fractures (McGowan 2003).

About 5 percent of fractures appear to be "spontaneous," in which the bone breaks first, then the person falls. The depleted bone mass and the structural deterioration of bone tissue leads to the weakening of bones. Osteoporosis may not cause a fall, but because of low-bone density, the risk of a fracture rises in affected individuals who experience a sudden strain or fall (Ott 2005).

Osteoporosis is a silent disease. Bones can become so fragile that they break under the slightest strain, without warning. People are often unaware that there frequently is a link between a fracture and osteoporosis. As a result, falls are especially dangerous for people who do not know that their bone density is low. This points out the necessity, particularly for women, to undergo a bone density test.

Fractures associated with osteoporosis are costly as well as debilitating. Few people are aware of how expensive bone disease can be for society and individuals with the disease. Care for fractures

---

Quick Facts about Falls and Fractures

- More than 90 percent of hip fractures are associated with osteoporosis.
- Nine out of ten hip fractures in older Americans are the result of a fall.
- Individuals who have a hip fracture are 5 to 20 percent more likely to die in the first year following an injury than others in this age group (sixty-five plus). Older adults who sustain a hip fracture are more likely to die in the first year than those who have not suffered hip fracture.
- For those living independently before a hip fracture, 15 to 25 percent will still be in long-term care institutions a year after their fracture.
- Most falls happen to women in their homes in the afternoon.

Source: NIAMS 2005

---

from osteoporosis costs Americans nearly $18 billion each year. Moreover, the cost of a hip fracture for one individual can be more than $81,000 overall (SG 2004). Osteoporosis is the most common cause of hip fractures, and prevention of this disease is fundamental to reducing the risk of hip fracture, especially in mature women (Genant et al. 1999; NIH 2002; NOF 1999). People are living longer, our elderly population is swelling, and the number of fractures will increase dramatically if precautions are not taken.

It has been shown that an adequate intake of calcium and vitamin D is necessary for the maintenance of adequate bone mass. Usually the diet of adults do not contain enough of these vital nutrients and therefore there is a great reliance on supplements to make up for any dietary deficiencies.

Figure 7.3. Calcium and Vitamin D Requirements

Age	Calcium (mg/day)	Vitamin D (IU— international units/day)
51–70 years	1,200	400
Over 70 years	1,200	600

(A cup of milk or fortified orange juice has about 300 mg of calcium and 50 IU of vitamin D.)

Source: National Academy of Sciences 1997

ADDITIONAL FACTORS THAT INCREASE FALL POTENTIAL

Falls in older adults are rarely attributed to one cause. Each year in the United States, nearly one-third of all older adults fall. In 2003, more than 13,700 people sixty-five years or older died of fall-related injuries. Nearly two million more were treated in emergency departments for nonfatal injuries related to falls. Given the growing population of this age group, the cost is expected to reach $43.8 billion by 2020 (CDC 2005).

While bone fragility is a major cause of falls, other factors come into play. Alterations in physical, emotional, and cognitive capacities markedly increase geriatric fall potential.

Medical and biological risk factors for falls vary widely, ranging from the effects of normal, healthy aging to pathological conditions commonly found in older adults. Typically, growing older includes reduced sensory, musculoskeletal, neurological, and metabolic function.

Women are three times more likely than men to be hospitalized for fall-related injuries. However, older men are 22 percent more likely than older women to die as the result of a fall. This may be because men sixty-five and older have more chronic conditions than women of the same age or because they engage in riskier behaviors, such as climbing on ladders or lifting heavy objects. Older adults who have fallen previously or who stumble frequently are two to three times more likely to fall within a year, as compared with older adults who have not fallen or do not slip or falter. Frail adults, those with impaired strength and balance, are three times more likely to fall as healthier persons of the same age, and they sustain more severe injuries when they do fall (CDC 2001).

Advanced age is also a factor that has long been associated with higher rates of falls. Seniors over eighty are the most likely to fall and be injured. The combined effects of an elderly individual's medical history play a very important part in estimating risks.

Muscle weakness and reduced physical fitness, particularly of the lower body, are typically considered widespread and inherent risk factors for falling. A combined panel of the American Geriatrics Society, British Geriatrics Society, and American Academy of Orthopaedic Surgeons found that this combination increases an elder's fall risk four to five times (AGS 2001). Furthermore, a loss of muscle strength, balance, flexibility, and coordination can also present dismaying obstacles to any older adult who is trying to complete the routine activities of daily living. Impaired mobility among older adults is an essential health consideration because if these circumstances cause them to become more and more sedentary, their fall risk rises sharply. The outcome of a fall, at that point, may very well be immobility and loss of independence.

Figure 7.4. Nonfatal Fall Injury Rates*

Year	Men	Women
2001	3,585.8	5,280.9
2002	3,482.7	5,233.4
2003	3,858.8	5,705.1
2004	3,850.6	5,719.9
2005	3,674.0	5,466.7

*Per 100,000 population; age adjusted to the 2000 US population.

Age-adjusted nonfatal fall injury rates among men and women age sixty-five years and older in the United States, 2001–2005. In 2005, the rate for women was almost 49 percent higher than for men.

Source: CDC 2005

Following are other prevalent factors that increase fall potential:

Acute Illnesses

Acute illness, such as a cold and its accompanying symptoms, may be responsible for between 10 and 20 percent of falls. One example is acute infection. Toxicity from infection can cause a change in mental status (Gleckman and Hibert 1982) and a confused, disoriented elderly adult is very likely to sustain a fall. A Canadian study suggested that people with infectious diseases are at a high risk for falls and injuries as a result of weakness, fatigue, or dizziness (Scott, Peck, and Kendall 2004).

Balance and Gait (Walking) Disorders

Factors such as dementia, instability, and fear of falling contribute to gait disorders. Inevitably, balance and gait disorders set the stage for the menacing deconditioning and coordination deficiencies that increase the risk for falling. However, as predictable as gait disorders are for contributing to falls and disability, healthcare providers generally agree that impaired gait may not be an unavoidable consequence of aging. Rather, it is very likely a manifestation of the increased prevalence of several age-associated diseases (Alexander 2005).

Health professionals are aware there are many active older adults who maintain a relatively normal gait pattern well into their eighties. Even so, all elders will experience at least a little slowing and a decrease in the length of their stride. These two factors are frequently mentioned in descriptions of gait disorders of the elderly.

Some researchers have referred to this age-related disorder as "essential senile gait disorder." The affected elder walks with legs wide apart, takes small steps, has a diminished arm swing and stooped posture, all of which lead to a tendency to fall. Although this disorder remains controversial, many clinicians feel that it may be a precursor to an undiagnosed disease or a symptom of coexisting, progressive cognitive impairment, for example, AD, vascular dementia, or normal pressure hydrocephalus (NPH) (Alexander 1999).

Even though medical and neurological challenges can cause gait abnormalities in older patients, healthcare providers also look at the obvious reasons why falls are so common in patients with dementia. Primarily, coordination is poor because of the individual's abnormal mental status. A leading symptom of dementia is poor judgment, and those who are cognitively impaired typically are unable to accurately assess their physical abilities, whether the action is as simple as trying to sit down in a chair or as complex as driving. Other contributing factors are the presence of osteoarthritis, which limits an individual's mobility, and the side effects of various medications that can suddenly heighten fall risks.

Impaired control of balance and gait is a leading factor in hastening instability and falls (Maki and McIlroy 2003). About 20 percent of community-dwelling older adults admit to having difficulty with walking, requiring the assistance of another person, or needing special equipment to help them walk. When equilibrium is a concern, the assessment of trunk sway can provide a simple way of reliably measuring changes in stability. This practice proves useful when screening for balance disorders of those prone to a fall (Gill et al. 2001). As an example, it is normal, during relaxed standing, for the body to sway continually—mostly backward and forward, with relatively little lateral sway. These movements are barely noticeable. But as people age, their postural sway increases, which in turn adds to their risk for falls.

Lack of Exercise/Sedentary Lifestyle

Most elders live a sedentary lifestyle. Another factor linked with falls is lack of exercise. Even though evidence continues to highlight the many benefits of exercise as a means of reducing the incidence of falls, it is often overlooked and underprescribed. Of special interest is the effectiveness of selected movements and drills, which when practiced on a regular basis produce a noticeable improvement in balance, mobility, and reaction time. Habitual fitness training has still another advantage: it also helps to increase bone mineral density in post-menopausal women and in all people age seventy and over.

Over the years, several research findings have demonstrated the efficacy of Tai Chi exercise in improving balance, reducing the risk of multiple falls, lessening the fear of falling, and improving ability to perform everyday tasks (Wolf et al. 1996; Kutner, Barnhart, and Wolf 1997). However, it is not clear whether this training can readily be implemented or adopted. In October 2005 the CDC funded a full prevention initiative to evaluate Tai Chi as a potential resource for elder communities (CDC 2007). As of this writing, researchers are observing adults sixty years and older who are physically mobile, with or without assistive devices, involved the Tai Chi program. They want to determine its effectiveness as a means of fall prevention and the practicality of introducing this program on a community-wide basis.

Balance Exercises to Do at Home

- Hold the back of a chair, sink, or countertop. Practice standing on one leg at a time for a minute. Gradually increase the time. Try balancing with eyes closed, then try without holding on.
- Hold the back of a chair, sink, or countertop. Practice standing on toes. Rock back to balance on heels. Hold each position for a count of ten.
- Hold the back of chair, sink, or countertop with both hands. Make a big circle to the left with hips; repeat to the right. Do not move shoulders or feet. Repeat five times.

Source: NIH Senior Health, http://www.nihseniorhealth.gov/osteoporosis/toc.html

Another beneficial resource for free booklets about exercises for older adults is found at http://www.niapublications.org/shopdisplay products.asp?id=30&cat=Healthy+Aging.

A comprehensive report released in 2003 concluded that exercise interventions reduced the risk of falls by 15 percent and the number of falls by 22 percent. Generally, fall-prevention exercise programs are designed to improve cardiovascular strength, muscle power, flexibility, and balance. Based on their findings, the researchers urge all older adults to participate in some general activity such as walking outside or mall walking indoors, cycling, mild aerobic movements, and other fitness activities including specific programs targeting increasing balance, strength, or flexibility (RAND 2003; Chang et al. 2004).

Vision Deficits

Changes in vision can precipitate a fall. Individuals with vision impairments—inability to adjust to light and darkness, altered depth perception, or reduced acuity—are about two and a half times more likely to incur a fall (AGS 2001).

In most cases diminished vision can be corrected with glasses, but changing prescriptions can take a while to get used to and can also contribute to a fall. The chances of this happening can be expected to rise if the glasses have new and unfamiliar multifocal lenses that alter depth perception (Eisenburg 2004). Some prescriptions may require glasses that are bifocal or trifocal. Consequently, when a person looks down through the lower half of the glasses, depth perception is altered. This impression can make it easy to lose balance and fall. To prevent this from happening, anyone who wears bi- or trifocals needs to practice looking straight ahead and lowering the head slightly in order to adjust to the changes that these lenses cause. Practicing at home or a familiar environment is recommended for safety reasons.

Reduced ability to adjust to light and darkness will also increase one's fall risk. In addition, as individuals mature, they may be susceptible to two of the leading causes of vision loss: macular degeneration and glaucoma. Because the risk of eye disease continues to increase with advancing age, everyone over sixty should be examined annually. More frequent examinations are recommended for adults with diabetes, hypertension, and other disorders, because these and many others can negatively affect vision.

Incontinence

Incontinence also increases an older adult's chances of falling. An accident usually occurs when a person rushes to the bathroom and does not take time to walk safely and assess the area for possible obstacles. Hazards are overlooked because the only thought in mind is getting to the toilet on time.

In healthcare settings, such as a hospital or a nursing home older, adults with urinary incontinence are also at increased risk of falling (Bakarich, McMillan, and Prosser 1997; Brown et al. 2001). For example, in hospitals falls occur during toileting activities, while in long-term care facilities falls occur in other locations, such as dining rooms, activity rooms, as well as bathrooms. Furthermore, residents report many occasions when they are unable to wait for staff assistance to get them to toilet facilities on time (Fleming et al. 1993).

An assessment that determines the type and severity of incontinence is an important component of any fall-prevention program for older adults. Older adults in long-term and acute care settings may benefit from a toileting program, as may older adults with functional and/or cognitive challenges (Bakarich, McMillan, and Prosser 1997).

Osteoarthritis

Although several chronic disorders are regularly linked to falls, particularly incontinence, cardiac arrhythmias, and stroke, acute illnesses also play a part, and they may be responsible for up to 20 percent of falls (Scott 2004).

Of the many chronic illnesses linked to falling, osteoarthritis is a leading example. It is a common chronic health condition of older adults in the United States (Verbrugge and Juarez 2001). Osteoarthritis is characterized by the breakdown of a joint's cartilage, the cushions at the ends of bones that allow easy movement of the joints. By age forty, almost everyone has some osteoarthritic changes in weight-bearing joints (for example, hip and knee joints) and, by age seventy-five, virtually everyone has some uncomfortable changes that limit activity in at least one joint. When present in the knee, osteoarthritis affects mobility, the ability to step over objects and maneuver, and the tendency to avoid complete weight bearing on a painful joint (Merck 2003).

Dementia occurs chiefly in elderly individuals, who almost certainly have some degree of osteoarthritis. However, it can be difficult to accurately assess their discomfort or pain because they may no longer be able to describe verbally how they feel. Some signs to look for are falling, increased agitation, tense muscles, bracing the body, and guarding extremities (Weissman 2000).

Polypharmacy

Medications can increase the probability of falls in older adults. Clinicians need to carefully evaluate the risks as well as the benefits of drug therapies given to those in their care. Many well-known medications have been associated with increased risk of falling, as well as starting on a new drug (Fuller 2004). Physical changes as people age increase the potential for adverse drug effects. And, although certain drugs may be known for their increased likelihood of side effects, the most prevalent cause for adverse drug reactions in later life is polypharmacy. The elderly consume a disproportionate quantity of drugs: on average, those sixty-five and older take two to six prescription and one to three nonprescription drugs at any one time (Routledge 2004).

Fortunately, the problems caused by polypharmacy are often readily correctable by modifying the types and amounts of drugs being taken. In most cases, informed families hold the key to averting their loved ones' harmful drug reactions and the potentially catastrophic consequences. Pharmacists, with their specialized skills, are trained to evaluate an individual's medication regimen for possible drug reactions that can lead to falls. These health professionals are in a key position to suggest medication modifications and educate patients and families on how to avoid potentially risky situations (Cooper et al. 1997). Both physician and pharmacist should be fully aware of what drugs, whether prescription or over-the-counter, are being taken.

It is always prudent to anticipate that all drugs have the potential for side effects and adverse reactions. Those who work in the health professions have a saying: "If it's strong enough to help you, it's strong enough to hurt you." It is good advice to follow.

Figure 7.5. Drugs Commonly Taken by Older Adults

Classification of Drugs Linked to Falls

Prescribed Drugs	**Over-the-Counter**
Analgesics	Alcohol
Antidepressants	Antacids
Antihypertensives	Laxatives
Anxiolytics	Nonsteroidal anti-inflammatory
Cardiovascular agents	agents
Diuretics	
Sedatives	
Tranquilizers	

PHYSICAL CHANGES THAT CONTRIBUTE TO ADVERSE DRUG EVENTS

Metabolism. The chemical processes that take place in the body's cells to convert fuel contained in food into energy are collectively known as metabolism. These chemical reactions are a constant function for all life-forms, and they exert major stress on the systems of the elderly body. As would be expected, the processes apply to medications as well as food, and sometimes pharmaceutical combinations can be toxic. When this happens, the results can be especially harmful for older adults.

Fat/water ratio. As people age they become "fattier." The body of an older adult has a reduced quantity of water and a larger relative amount of fat than that of someone younger. Therefore, the amount of a drug per pound of body weight or per pound of water will often measure higher in elders than the same dosage given to younger patients. Furthermore, since an older adult has proportionately more body fat, drugs that collect in fat tissue are more likely to remain in the body longer because there is more fat in which they can accumulate.

Liver function. Although the liver undergoes several age-related changes in terms of its structure and function, it still performs fairly well in old age. Some changes include a decrease in liver size and a reduction in the flow of blood and bile. It is difficult to estimate hepatic clearance in older adults for several reasons. The effects of aging, concurrent illnesses, and drug classification will all influence the amount of a drug or drugs that will be removed from the body by the liver. Surprisingly, the evidence from newer research shows that there is little difference between ninety-year-olds and younger individuals when comparing results of some liver function tests (Schmucker 2001).

There have been numerous drug–liver function investigations over the years, and the best recommendation still seems to be the familiar warning when prescribing medications: "start lower, go slower." This advice is more pertinent than ever due to the amount of new drugs entering the marketplace. This warning especially applies to drugs that affect the kidneys and liver. General recommendations are to use a starting dose that is 30 to 40 percent smaller than the average dose used for middle-aged adults (Zeeh and Platt 2002).

Renal (kidney) function. The kidneys are vital organs that perform many functions to keep the blood chemically balanced. Blood is filtered by the kidneys. The actual filtering occurs in units within the kidneys called *nephrons*. As people age, however, the kidneys diminish in size and gradually become less efficient at removing waste products from the blood. Decreases in renal blood flow have been approximated at 10 percent per decade beginning after age forty (Mühlberg and Platt 1999).

The primary reason renal disease is so common in elderly individuals is because of the chronic effects of hypertension. According to the National Center for Health Statistics, 50 million adults in the United States, including more than half of those over sixty, have high blood pressure (NIH 2002).

Alcohol

It may be surprising to learn that as much as 15 percent of older adults who live independently in the community are considered problem drinkers (SAMHSA 2007). Furthermore, the numbers are even higher among older adults seen in different healthcare settings (doctors' offices, hospitals) and in residents of nursing homes (Callahan and Tierney 1995; Friedmann et al. 1999).

Excessive drinking generally results in symptoms of memory loss, confusion, disorientation, and imbalance. Even drinking a small amount of alcohol can impair judgment, coordination, and reaction time. In older adults, drinking often increases household accidents, including falls resulting in hip fractures.

Facts at a Glance

- As many as 3 million people sixty and over in the United States have a problem with alcohol.
- Widowers over seventy-five have the highest rate of alcoholism in the country.
- In 1991 an estimated 70 percent of hospital admissions of older people were for alcohol-related problems.
- Physicians miss a diagnosis of alcoholism or fail to record the information on their elderly patients nearly half of the time.

Community surveys indicate hazardous and harmful alcohol consumption patterns are prevalent among older adults (Adams 1996; Moore and O'Keeffe 1999). These individuals are often able to conceal their risky behavior from family, friends, and physicians. Also, an estimated 19 percent of older Americans may be affected by combined difficulties with alcohol and medication misuse.

The effects of alcohol vary with age. Slower reaction times, problems with hearing and seeing, and a lower tolerance to alcohol's effects put older people at higher risk for falls and other types of injuries.

Mixing alcohol with over-the-counter or prescription medications can be very dangerous, even fatal. Problems with alcohol intensify most medical conditions common in older people, such as hypertension, depression, and ulcers. Elderly individuals react differently than younger adults because of the physical changes associated with aging. An old person can feel "high" even after drinking only small amounts of alcohol. Therefore, even if there is no medical reason to avoid alcohol, older men and women should limit themselves to one drink per day.

It is important to remember that alcohol is a drug. Moreover, it is classified as a depressant and it slows brain activity. As a general rule, it is typically unsafe to mix it with medications. More than 150 medications are known to interact harmfully with alcohol, resulting in increased risk of illness, injury, and even death.

Alcohol's effects are heightened by medicines that depress the central nervous system, such as sleeping pills, antihistamines, antidepressants, anti-anxiety drugs, and some painkillers. In addition, medicines for certain disorders, including diabetes, high blood pressure, and heart disease, can have dangerous interactions with alcohol. Anyone who is taking an over-the-counter or prescription medication needs to ask a physician or pharmacist if drinking alcohol is contraindicated or inadvisable.

FALL-PREVENTION STRATEGIES

People who have already fallen, even if they weren't injured, tend to develop an almost abnormal fear of falling. They lose confidence, hesitate at the wrong time, lose their balance, and fall again. Preoccupation with the fear often generates other negative effects: it causes individuals to limit their activities, which soon leads to reduced mobility, increased isolation, increased sedentary behavior, and an escalating fall risk (Vellas et al. 1997).

The data suggest a bleak outlook, but the many practical strategies we've covered can be implemented in order to avoid becoming a statistic. Fall prevention is the first line of defense. It is both practical and beneficial to have an occupational therapist come in and assess the home of anyone who is at high risk for slips, trips, and falls (Cumming, Thomas, and Szonyi 1999). The occupational therapist may also recommend to the patient or caregiver various mechanical devices for easing the burden in daily living activities at this time.

Resources for Mobility Aids and Assistive Technology

- Technology products and rehabilitation equipment available from domestic and international sources, online at http://www.abledata.com.
- Information about lifting equipment, online at http://www.aema.com/accessibility_equipment.html.

MORBIDITY AND MORTALITY

Stays are almost twice as long for elderly patients who are hospitalized after a fall than for those who are admitted for other reasons (Dunn et al. 1992). Moreover, if dementia is an issue, the patient's susceptibility to complications increase. Incontinence, urinary tract infections, pneumonia, bed sores, and malnutrition are just a few of the developing disorders associated with longer hospital stays.

The mortality rate for falls increases dramatically with age in both sexes. Statistics show that 70 percent of accidental deaths in persons seventy-five and older are caused by falls. Furthermore, over 90 percent of hip fractures occur as a result of falls, with most of these fractures occurring in persons over seventy, and nearly a fourth of hip fracture patients die within a year of their injury (Leibson et al. 2002).

Age, vision and hearing deficits, and medications heighten every older adult's fall risk. When dementia is an additional factor, the chances of falling increase greatly.

Chapter 8
Advice and Consent

As people with dementia near the end stages of their disease, they do not often receive the best care. Pain control is frequently inadequate, and patients may be subjected to invasive and ineffective treatments (Sachs 2004). Families can help avoid these distressing and unnecessary problems through advance planning.

In ideal situations, older adults have planned and made decisions in advance for emergencics. They have assessed future living arrangements, made informed choices about life-sustaining medical care, and ensured that documents, instructions, and powers of attorney are available to those who must take responsibility if a crisis occurs.

When an individual develops Alzheimer's or any other dementia, families generally arc thrust into roles for which they are unprepared. As examples, they may suddenly need to arrange for a home health aide to help with personal care, plan for nursing home placement, or deal with end-of-life decisions. These demands are emotionally and physically stressful.

One of the most difficult tasks for a family member is having to make medical, legal, or financial decisions on behalf of a loved one who is seriously ill without having a complete understanding of the individual's preferences. In order to avoid the frustration and anxiety that are bound to occur in such situations, older adults need to discuss their end-of-life wishes with family members and healthcare providers well before the onset of a serious illness. It also is equally important to designate a surrogate decision maker for healthcare at this time.

PATIENT SELF-DETERMINATION ACT

As most are aware, the capabilities to prolong life have improved substantially as drug development and medical technology have advanced. Nevertheless, this has proved to be a mixed blessing since medical intervention may only prolong discomfort in end-of-life situations.

In order to protect an individual's right to either accept or refuse specific medical or surgical care, Congress passed the Patient Self-Determination Act (PSDA), which became effective in 1991. As a result, patient involvement in decisions about life-sustaining treatments while they were still competent to do so became greater than ever before. The act requires hospitals, skilled nursing facilities, and other healthcare settings to develop written policies and give patients clear information concerning advance directives, including do-not-resuscitate (DNR) orders (AHRQ 2003). The PSDA further requires that institutions document relevant patient information and verify that directives are in each individual's chart.

Essentially, the act requires most healthcare institutions (but not individual doctors) do the following:

- Provide patients upon admission with a written summary of an individual's health care decision-making rights and the facility's policies with respect to recognizing advance directives.
- Ask patients if they have an advance directive and document whether they do in the medical record. It is the patient's responsibility to provide the facility with a copy.
- Educate the staff about advance directives (ABA 2007).

ADVANCE CARE PLANNING

Patients have the right to decide ahead of time what kind of treatment they do or do not want if hospitalized and unable to speak for themselves. Advance care planning is a process that helps to accomplish this by preparing for end-of-life concerns. This is done by means of a written statement called an advance directive. In it a person lists specific end-of-life treatment preferences, a living will, and a durable power of attorney for healthcare, also called a healthcare proxy (Poncy 2006).

Trying to anticipate what kind of treatment patients will want at the end of life is complicated by several factors: age, nature of the illness, ability of medicine to sustain life, and emotions that families experience when a loved one is sick and may be dying. Advance directives are simple legal documents specifically authorized by state laws that allow patients to make their health preferences known and that provide instructions for care in case they become incapacitated and cannot make decisions for themselves (AHRQ 2003).

Critically ill patients and their families struggle with powerful life-altering questions. Initially they need to decide whether to continue treatment. If the choice is to continue, other questions come in to play. For example, how intensive is the therapy and how long will it be used? Families also want to understand the risks involved and the potential benefits, side effects, and alternative treatments. In these situations, patients rely on physicians, nurses, spiritual advisers, and other trusted professionals for guidance. Advance care planning can help prevent loved ones from being forced to make decisions in ignorance or in a crisis situation.

Spiritual, religious, and cultural beliefs may have a bearing on the types of advance directives one chooses to prepare. Although death is typically a difficult subject to bring up, the only way to ensure that everyone understands the patient's values and beliefs is to discuss them ahead of time.

THE LIVING WILL

The living will is a legal document that expresses a person's wishes about medical treatment at the end of life (AA 2008). The document is used if an individual becomes terminally ill, incapacitated, or unable to communicate or make decisions about medical care intended to sustain life. It should be as specific as possible, detailing the amount of care a patient wants while he or she is unable to make a decision, for example, in a coma situation.

Well-publicized court cases, notably those of Nancy Cruzan and Terri Schiavo, have furthered widespread general interest in planning for healthcare choices. Another law with comprehensive features facilitating advance directives is the Uniform Health Care Decisions Act (UHCDA) of 1993. This act also addresses the issues of decision making for those who have failed to plan (English 2001). The full text of the UHCDA is available online at http://www.nccusl.org.

> Living wills are not yet legally enforceable in Massachusetts, Michigan, and New York (English 2001). However, healthcare proxies are legal documents, recognized in all fifty states (Stern 2006).

Not everyone understands that accepting or refusing medical care is a patient's right. The living will, with its documented instructions about medical care intended to prolong life, reaffirms this right. The living will also removes the burden for making decisions from family, friends, and physicians.

There are many types of life-sustaining care that need to be addressed when drafting a living will. Some of the topics that ought to be included are:

- The use of life-sustaining equipment (dialysis machines, ventilators, and respirators)

- Do not resuscitate (DNR) orders, instructions not to use cardiopulmonary resuscitation (CPR) if breathing or heartbeat stops
- Artificial hydration and nutrition (tube feeding)
- Withholding of food and fluids
- Palliative/comfort care
- Organ and tissue donation

It is essential that everyone understands that a decision not to receive "aggressive medical treatment" (sometimes referred to as "heroic measures") is not the same as withholding all medical care. For example, patients can still receive pain medication, antibiotics, nutrition, radiation therapy, and other interventions when the goal of treatment becomes comfort rather than cure. This is called *palliative care*, and its primary focus is on pain relief and helping the patient remain as comfortable as possible.

Patients can also change their minds and ask their physicians to resume more aggressive treatment. If the type of treatment a patient would like to receive changes, however, it is important to be aware that such a decision may raise insurance issues and the patient's medical insurance plan will need to be reviewed. Any changes in the type of treatment a patient wants to receive need to be reflected in the patient's living will.

A durable power of attorney for healthcare is an advance directive in which an individual names someone else (the agent, or proxy) to make healthcare decisions in the event the individual becomes unable to make them. A patient should be sure to ask this person for agreement to act as an agent. Instructions may also be included about any treatments that individual wants to avoid.

A durable power of attorney for finances is a legal document that gives someone authority to manage another individual's finances should that person become incapacitated. This is usually an agent or an attorney-in-fact (Nolo 2008). This is a separate legal document from the durable power of attorney for healthcare. Patients may choose the same person or someone besides their healthcare proxy to act as agent in financial matters.

> To find your state's approved forms, click on your state's official Web site and type "advance directive" in search box.
> Other sources include healthcare providers, state medical societies, state health departments, and legal offices.

It is important to understand that advance directives are for everyone of legal age, not just older adults. The whole process of planning now for death is a considerate and clear-cut way for a person to express concern, thoughtfulness, and love for family and friends. Prompt preparation allows them to know clearly, and without equivocation, a loved one's wishes, particularly since the survivors will be the ones faced with the difficult and painful decisions. It also helps to reduce the possibility of friction among family members or guilty feelings that frequently cause difficulties in such situations.

Decisions about types of treatment will always have implications for costs, care, and use of scarce medical resources. Finally, the entire preparation process can be a meaningful experience that contributes to the spiritual growth of both patients and families.

Methods for advance medical planning were originally developed to ensure that patients' preferences would guide the nature and intensity of their future medical care.

The directives were developed because people gradually became aware that the initial goals of medical technology and the pharmaceutical industry to make lives better could also be used in ways that seemed uncertain, confusing, and even self-serving and harmful.

The purpose of advance directives is to allay fears and concerns. In the past, there have been traumatic events that resulted in end-of-life situations where the care and treatment of the patient appeared to be excessive, ineffective, and distressingly burdensome to patients and their families. The protracted, glaring publicity of certain high-profile court cases—notably of Karen Ann Quinlan in 1976 (Hyland and Baime 1976), Nancy Cruzan in 1990 (Momeyer 1990), and more recently Terri Schiavo in 2005 (Ulferts et al. 2005)—are examples of what might happen when no advance directive is written or available. The litigation called attention to the importance of leaving unambiguous instructions about treatment preferences to be honored if an individual becomes incapacitated. It also stresses the importance of appointing a trusted alternate or proxy to make medical decisions for an individual who is no longer able to do so. The development of advance directives was an outgrowth of the Quinlan case. The recent Schiavo case has led to renewed interest in living wills.

Ideally, patients, families, and physicians hold discussions about treatment options that include the length and invasiveness of treatment, chances of success, overall prognosis, and the quality of life during and after treatment. The talks should be ongoing, reflecting changes in the patient's situation. Unfortunately, families too often do not have such conversations among themselves or with their healthcare providers. Trying to second-guess what a demented person would have wanted is the least desirable way of addressing the problem of continued medical treatment.

Patients' end-of-life preferences are highly individualized and influenced largely by personal beliefs that cannot be assumed or predicted (Donaldson and Field 1998). There is ample evidence suggesting although most patients have not participated in advance care planning, it does not mean they are not willing to discuss end-of-life care. Often they wait until their physicians initiate discussions. One way to determine patients' preferences for end-of-life care is to discuss hypothetical situations and find out their opinions on certain treatment patterns. These opinions can help clarify and predict their preferences if they should become unable to make their own decisions.

Instructions for an Advance Directive

1. Choose two people—a healthcare agent and an alternate.
2. Discuss your wishes with your agent, the alternate, your family, and your primary care physician, or even your spiritual adviser or attorney.
3. Complete your statement of wishes (living will).
4. Give copies of the healthcare proxy and the living will to people named in 2.
5. Do not keep the only copy in your safe deposit box.

END-OF-LIFE DECISIONS

One of the most difficult decisions for anyone to make is to predict what treatments a loved one will want at the end of life. End of life has only recently commanded the attention of public health officials, even though its significance as one of society's major health concerns is widely recognized. The myriad choices available are inevitably complicated by the patient's age, the nature of illness, the ability of medicine to sustain life, and the emotions that the families must endure when their loved ones are sick and possibly dying.

Much of the suffering that is often a component of terminal illness—whether physical or mental—can be readily managed. However, the more effective strategies and interventions are not always accessible to everyone. As an example, studies point to disparities in hospice use, particularly among patients with certain types of cancer, such as prostate cancer. It is unclear whether these disparities are due to lack of awareness regarding the options for end-of-life care or to differences in perspectives regarding the end of life (CDC 2007).

Most people will find it difficult to talk about end-of-life issues. Nevertheless, even though discussions of the subject may be uncomfortable, having these conversations is the best way to protect one's independence in countless unpredictable situations. Fortunately, there are resources available that can help encourage meaningful conversations and practical planning for end-of-life care.

End of life is very often linked to significant suffering among dying individuals and also imposes health and financial consequences that affect family members as well as society. The data indicate that as many as 50 percent of dying persons with cancer or other chronic illnesses experience unrelieved symptoms during their final days. Moreover, recent studies demonstrate an increased likelihood of depressive symptoms and mortality among the caregivers of terminally ill patients (CDC 2007).

About a quarter of all hospitalized patients are treated in intensive care or cardiac care units before they die, and more Americans die in hospitals than anywhere else (Kaufman 2005). End-of-life care has been acknowledged as an important clinical issue needing improvement. There is compelling evidence demonstrating that advance planning can effectively guide end-of-life decisions (Hammes and Rooney 1998).

Public health strategies and medical treatment advances have been so effective that they resulted in a thirty-year increase in life expectancy during the twentieth century. More to the point, as people are living longer their expectations about quality of life, including at its very end, are increasing. Seventy-eight percent of Americans live past their sixty-fifth birthday, and more than three-fourths of them will have to contend with cancer, stroke, heart disease, obstructive lung disease, or dementia during their last years of life (Lynn 2000).

Chronic conditions—illnesses that last longer than three months—are the leading cause of disability and death in the United States. As the population ages, the incidence of such conditions will increase. However, it is misleading to think that chronic conditions primarily affect the elderly. Two-thirds of chronically ill people are under sixty-five. By 2020, chronic conditions are projected to afflict approximately 157 million people, about half of US population. Currently there are about 120 million chronic disease sufferers (AHCJ 2002).

Naturally, death will prevail, and most people will die as a result of a chronic condition. The public health field is aware of this issue and plays a critical role in helping Americans maintain quality of life throughout their lives.

Resources for End-of-Life Care

- Caring Conversations is a consumer education initiative that helps individuals and their families share meaningful conversation while making practical preparations for end-of-life decisions, available online at http://www .practicalbioethics.org.
- Caring Connections is a program of the National Hospice and Palliative Care Organization that can be accessed at http://www.caringinfo.org.
- *Finding Your Way: A Guide for Medical Decisions Near the End of Life*, is a thirteen-page booklet available in English and Spanish that was developed in response to the concerns of healthcare professionals and consumers. This booklet may be ordered online at http:// www.sachealthdecisions.org/finding.html.
- For general information about home care, the National Association for Home Care and Hospice (NAHC) currently distributes helpful booklets to consumers. An example is "All about Hospice: A Consumer's Guide." NAHC serves as a clearinghouse for home care and hospice facts and statistics. The Web site is http://www .nahc.org.
- The Family Caregiver Alliance at http://www.caregiver .org/caregiver/jsp/home.jsp is another useful resource. Individuals can find out what services are available in their state simply by using the above Web site and navigating to the tab that says "Caregiving Info and Advice" to find what services their state offers.

> • For guardianship/surrogacy issues and protection of elders, consumers need to go their states' Web sites, which can be accessed by using http://www.statelocal gov.net and clicking on the state in question; then scroll down to "Executive Branch" and locate the Department of Elder Affairs or Department of Senior Services to find the local Area Agency on Aging. It is through that agency that protective services can be reached and inquiries made.

EMERGENCY MEDICAL TECHNICIANS, DO NOT RESUSCITATE ORDERS, AND COMFORT CARE

Emergency medical technicians (EMTs) and paramedics are required to provide emergency care to the fullest extent possible and transport patients to appropriate healthcare facilities. However, there is an exception to this imperative.

More and more patients are choosing not to be resuscitated when medical options are extremely limited and their quality of life is deteriorating. Comfort care targets pain management. Patients who will refuse resuscitation efforts may direct their physicians to prepare a formal order that permits only comfort measures. The directive is called a Comfort Care/DNR Order, and it allows EMTs and first responders to honor a DNR order in an out-of-hospital setting in many states. People are urged to ask their individual healthcare providers about the Comfort Care/DNR forms and/or bracelets.

PALLIATIVE CARE/HOSPICE CARE

For the past several decades, the healthcare system has provided a number of options to ease the dying experience. Medical treatment has expanded to include palliative care and hospice care. The goal of palliative care is to achieve an optimal quality of life for patients by using a holistic approach that focuses on symptoms, alleviation of pain, and the other unique needs of a patient with a serious or life-threatening illness. A combination of social support, emotional support, and attention to spiritual aspects of care and respect for the patient's culture, beliefs, and values are essential components of this approach.

Although the level of palliative care intensifies at the end of life, focus on the relief of suffering and improvement of quality of life is important throughout the course of the illness, and aspects of palliative care can be provided along with life-prolonging treatment during earlier phases of a patient's illness. Having a patient live with dignity during this hard time is key, and it is the mission of an interdisciplinary team of specially trained health professionals and volunteers to achieve this.

Hospice care is delivered to dying patients in inpatient units, nursing homes, or, most often, in their own homes. Along with pain control and symptom management, emotional and spiritual support is provided. Hospice is generally available around the clock, seven days a week. In addition to providing palliative care and personal encouragement to individuals at the end of their lives, hospice also meets the psychosocial needs of the family during this difficult time as well as during the bereavement period.

In 1982 Medicare began reimbursing certified Medicare hospices that are in hospitals, home health agencies, and nursing homes for hospice services. In order to qualify for the Medicare hospice benefit, patients must have a terminal diagnosis, a life-expectancy of six months or less, and must be willing to forgo further treatment. Patients who live longer than six months can be "recertified" if their situation still meets the criteria for the benefit (CDC 2007).

Cancer remains the most common primary diagnosis for those using hospice. However, patients with other terminal illnesses such as heart disease, dementia, cerebrovascular disease, and chronic obstructive pulmonary disease also qualify for hospice. Although the hospice benefit provides integrated care services, prescription medications, and counseling for patients and family members, it is underutilized by Medicare beneficiaries with Alzheimer's disease (HHS 2000).

WHO PAYS FOR HOSPICE?

The following are examples of the primary sources of payment for hospice care:

- Private insurance or personal or family assets: private health insurance, for example, a health maintenance organization (HMO); Social Security (including Supplemental Security Income); retirement funds; or welfare, among others. It does not include Veterans Administration (VA) contracts, pensions, or other VA compensation.
- Medicare, a federal program, is the nation's largest health insurer for people sixty-five and over. Coverage is also extended to some disabled people under sixty-five and people with end-stage renal disease (permanent kidney failure treated with dialysis or a transplant). Under the Medicare program funds are received for home health or hospice care and may be obtained through fee-for-service Medicare or Medicare HMO. For a more complete description about Medicare hospice benefits, visit http://www.cms.hhs.gov.
- Medicaid provides medical assistance for certain individuals and families with low incomes and few resources. Medicaid is funded by money given to the state by the federal government under the Medicaid Program for home health or hospice care. It may be obtained through fee-for-service Medicaid or Medicaid HMO. Each state has its own eligibility requirements for receiving benefits. Although the federal government sets general guidelines for the program, Medicaid eligibility is determined by each state. More specific information can be found at http://www.cms.hhs.gov.

- An older adult who receives Medicare benefits and who has a modest income may be eligible for the Qualified Medicare Beneficiary program. If the individual qualifies, the state he lives in will pay the Medicare premiums, deductibles, and co-insurance. Families who think their loved one may qualify need to contact their local medical assistance (Medicaid) agency, social services office, or welfare office for information.

- Medicare provides basic healthcare coverage, but it does not pay all medical expenses, nor does it pay for most long-term care. For this reason, many private companies sell insurance to fill the gaps in Medicare coverage. This kind of insurance is generally referred to as Medigap insurance. Contact the Health Care Financing Administration's Medigap Hotline toll free at 1-800-638-6833 for more information.

- For more help with Medicare questions, call 1-800-MEDICARE. For the speech and hearing impaired, call TTY/TDD: 1-877-486-2048. Further information is available at www.medicare.gov. Other sources include religious organizations; foundations; Veterans Administration contracts, pensions, or other VA compensation; and other military medical programs.

ARE DOCUMENTED PREFERENCES EVER IGNORED?

Although the goal of advance directives is to make certain patients receive treatment that is consistent with their preferences, there are no guarantees that this will be the case. Moreover, there is ample evidence indicating that the well-meaning efforts on the parts of patients, families, physicians, and legal teams may go unrecognized (Teno et al. 1997). When and if this happens, it is possible that patients may receive care that conflicts with their previously expressed wishes (Hanson, Tulsky, and Danis 1997).

Advance directives are overlooked for a variety of reasons: documents may be forgotten at the time of hospital admission, they may be improperly filed or stored, or they may be inaccessible, for example, when the sole copy is left in a safe deposit box (Broadwell et al. 1993; Morrison et al. 1995). In addition, emergency medical services may not have tangible evidence that enables them to recognize DNR orders in an out-of-hospital setting.

The problem may not be the content of advance directives, but rather the way in which healthcare professionals act on them. For example, physicians may be hesitant to initiate discussions about advance directives with patients, especially early in the course of an illness (Shojania et al. 2001). Doctors have also indicated that time pressure can be an obstacle, thereby defeating efforts to promote following advance directives among their elderly primary care patients (Wissow et al. 2004).

Advance directives are open to subjective interpretation. Much of this ambiguity is related to the vagueness of the directive's terminology, whereas in other instances it may be traced to the tendency for health professionals to make value judgments based on their own feelings concerning quality-of-life issues (Thompson, Barbour, and Schwartz 2003).

Although a lawyer is not needed to complete an advance directive, it is important to be aware that each state has its own laws for creating advance directives. These laws vary from state to state and should be noted wherever the patient lives or is treated.

This does not mean, however, that advance directives or advance care planning is futile or unnecessary. Despite their shortcomings, advance directives remain the best available approach for helping patients plan future care.

Families need to constantly monitor their loved one's care. They can do so through personal research, critical questioning, and frequent discussion with the healthcare providers involved. Having current information is an essential component in making sound healthcare decisions. In the end, no legal document can replace prudent, caring choices that are made promptly when the treatment dilemma is clear.

ADDRESSING END-OF-LIFE ISSUES

Major advances in public health and medicine have shifted the leading cause of death from infectious disease to chronic disease; Americans no longer die from influenza outbreaks, per se, but from the lingering effects of cancer. As a result, most people alive today will die at an advanced age following a period of chronic illness. At the same time, with innovations in medical technology and treatment protocols, quality of life and of dying have become increasingly important issues for the general public.

A significant but often overlooked end-of-life concern is the health of the caregiver. Typically, elderly individuals with cognitive impairments are cared for by a spouse or an adult child. It has been well known for some time that these caregivers sustain increased rates of depression and other serious illnesses. Less well publicized is the rise in mortality rates of these individuals (Shultz and Beach 1999). *The State of Aging and Health in America 2007*, a report released by the CDC, reaffirms these public health risks and warns of the health and economic consequences to Americans (CDC 2007). Meeting these challenges is essential so that baby boomers can look forward to their own "golden years." More than a third of US deaths are preventable and three behaviors—smoking, poor diet, and physical inactivity—were the root causes of almost 35 percent of US deaths in 2000. These behaviors are the ones that often underlie the development of the nation's leading chronic disease killers, which are heart disease, cancer, stroke, and diabetes.

DEATH AND DECISIONS

When a loved one dies, grieving family members are immediately confronted with numerous difficult choices and decisions when everyone is under extreme emotional pressure. A few of the immediate questions survivors will need to answer are:

- Should there be burial or cremation?
- Will there be a religious service?
- Is the deceased an organ donor?
- Which funeral provider will be used?
- Are there mandatory products or services survivors need to buy?

Furthermore, as insensitive as it may sound at the time, virtually everyone wonders how much things will cost and how they will be paid for.

Each year Americans struggle with these and many other questions as they spend billions of dollars arranging funerals for family members or friends. The increasing trend toward preplanning suggests that many consumers want to compare prices and services so that ultimately the funeral reflects a carefully researched and well-informed purchasing decision. Prudent consumers review and revise their plans periodically (FTC 2007).

WHAT IS THE FUNERAL RULE AND HOW CAN IT HELP CONSUMERS?

Most funeral service providers are principled professionals who look out for the best interests of the consumer. However, not all are ethical vendors. The Funeral Rule is a federal law developed by the Federal Trade Commission (FTC) that was enacted by Congress in 1982. This law requires funeral directors to give anyone who asks an itemized general price list for their goods and services. It also requires funeral directors to be informative and unambiguous.

Even simple funerals can be an expensive purchase for many consumers. A traditional funeral, including a casket and vault, costs about six thousand dollars, although extras like flowers, obituary notices, acknowledgment cards, or limousines can add thousands of dollars to the bill. It is not uncommon for funerals to exceed ten thousand dollars.

Below is a checklist for consumers to use when visiting funeral homes and comparing costs.

Funerals: A Consumer Guide

Simple disposition of the remains
Immediate burial
Immediate cremation
If the cremation process is extra, how much is it?
Donation of the body to a medical school

Traditional, full-service burial or cremation
Basic services fee for the funeral director and staff
Pickup of body
Embalming
Other preparation of body
Least expensive casket
Description, including model number
Outer burial container (vault)
Description
Visitation/viewing—staff, facilities
Funeral or memorial service—staff, facilities
Graveside service
Hearse
Other
Total

Other services
Forwarding body to another funeral home
Receiving body from another funeral home

Cemetery/mausoleum costs
Cost of lot or crypt (if you do not already own one)
Perpetual care
Opening or closing grave or crypt
Grave liner, if required
Marker, monument (including setup)

Source: FTC 2007

The Federal Trade Commission's brochure for consumers titled "Funerals: A Consumer Guide" provides additional information about consumers' rights and legal requirements when planning funerals. The commission also offers a free handbook for funeral providers titled "Complying with the Funeral Rule." Information is available at the FTC Web site, http://www.ftc.gov, and from the Consumer Response Center, Room 130, 600 Pennsylvania Avenue NW, Washington, DC, 20580, or call toll free 1-877-FTC-HELP.

> The FTC has an online complaint form at https://rn.ftc .gov/pls/dod/wsolcq$.startup?Z_ORG_CODE=PU01. Consumers can also call 1-877-FTC-HELP.

Consumers need to be aware that there are people who unhesitatingly take advantage of recently bereaved older adults. For instance, a banker pled guilty to embezzlement, admitting he took a total of $360,859.04 deposited by six different clients. He stole the money by closing or depleting CD and IRA accounts belonging to the victims and deposited the funds into his personal account. He then attempted to conceal his fraud by forging withdrawal slips and destroying bank surveillance tapes. All the victims were elderly. The youngest victim was seventy-three, the oldest, ninety-two. He targeted couples where one spouse had recently passed away.

Obituaries often contain personal information that captures the attention of unscrupulous individuals. Consequently, lawyers and business advocates suggest that families devise a strategy for handling claims on a loved one's estate before an obituary appears in the local newspaper.

VETERANS' CEMETERIES

All veterans are entitled to a free burial in a national cemetery and a grave marker. This eligibility also extends to some civilians who have provided military-related service and some US Public Health Service personnel. Spouses and dependent children of veterans also are entitled to a lot and marker when buried in a national cemetery.

There are no charges for opening or closing the grave, for a vault or liner, or for setting the marker in a national cemetery. Typically, the family is responsible for other expenses, including transportation to the cemetery. For more information, visit the Department of Veterans Affairs Web site at www.cem.va.gov. To reach the regional veterans office in your area, call 1-800-827-1000.

The US Department of Veterans Affairs provides valuable information for veterans and their survivors on such topics as eligibility for burial benefits and burial allowance at http://www.cem.va.gov.

HELPING WITH A FRAIL ELDER'S BUSINESS AFFAIRS

There may come a time when a family member or trusted friend needs to step in and help a frail elderly individual manage legal and financial responsibilities. The person who takes on the tasks typically has scant knowledge of the elder's vital information and records. This may cause valuable time to be wasted not only during the elder's lifetime but especially after death. Advanced preparation avoids the unnecessary anxiety and stress suffered when important documents or household records are needed and cannot be located.

The following sample forms may serve as guides for caregivers and help them to tailor suitable documents for their own needs.

Figure 8.1. Sample Personal Records File

Personal records file for _____

For a quick reference, check the box next to items on hand and note location.

❏ Birth certificate
❏ Certificates of marriage, divorce, citizenship
❏ Names and addresses of spouse and children (location of death certificates, if applicable)
❏ Prearrangement for burial
❏ Social Security number
❏ Will or trust
❏ Living will
❏ Durable power of attorney for healthcare
❏ Life insurance
❏ Accident insurance
❏ Health insurance
❏ Pension plan(s)
❏ Bank account(s)
❏ Tax returns
❏ Safe deposit box(es)
❏ Car(s)
❏ Real estate/rental papers
❏ Others (citizenship papers, education and military records, etc.)

_____
_____

Personal Inventory

Name _____
Date _____
Address _____
Date and Place of Birth _____
Social Security Number _____

Next of Kin

Name _____
Address _____
Employer _____
Name _____
Address _____
Benefits _____

Personal Papers (birth certificates, living will, etc.)
Location _____

Insurance Companies _____

Life (name and policy number)

_____

Automobile (name and policy number)

_____

Other (name and policy number)

_____

Banking Papers (include pension plans, if any)

Kind of account, bank name/address, account number
_____

Kind of account, bank name/address, account number
_____

Other accounts (include pension plans and safe deposit boxes)
_____
_____

     Where _____

     Account number _____

Automobile(s) (make, model, year) _____

Real estate papers __ _____

Personal items of value
_____
_____
_____

Professionals who can help with my personal and business affairs

Attorney _____

Insurance agent _____

Doctor _____

Clergy _____

Other (broker, business colleague, accountant)
_____
_____
_____

Funeral arrangements

_____

_____

_____

_____

_____

Special requests

_____

_____

_____

_____

The National Center for Health Statistics maintains a Web site for copies of vital records such as birth, death, marriage and divorce at http://www.cdc.gov/nchs/howto/w2w/w2welcom.htm.

The IRS has a program called Tax Counseling for the Elderly (TCE) that offers free tax help for individuals sixty or older, available online at http://www.irs.gov/individuals/article/0,,id=109754,00.html.

The IRS also has other programs that offer free assistance with tax return preparation and tax-filing volunteers trained by IRS partners. For more information on the times and locations of assistance or to learn how to become a volunteer, call the IRS at 1-800-829-1040 or go to http://www.aarp.org/money/taxaide.

Figure 8.2. Sample Financial Records File

When making a financial records file, list information about insurance policies, bank accounts, deeds, investments, and other valuables, using this outline:

- Sources of income and assets (pension funds, interest income, etc.)
- Social Security and Medicare information
- Investment income (stocks, bonds, and property)
- Insurance information (life, health, and property) with policy numbers
- Bank accounts (checking, savings, credit union)
- Location of safe deposit boxes
- Copy of most recent income tax return
- Liabilities: what is owed to whom and when payments are due
- Mortgages and debts: how and when paid
- Credit card and charge account names and numbers
- Property taxes
- Location of valuable personal items such as jewelry, antiques, etc.

THE IMPORTANCE OF A WILL

A will is document that is of great significance because it provides people with the means of giving instructions about the distribution of their money and property when they die. In it, the testator (the person who makes a will) names an executor to carry out the testator's instructions. An executor may be a trusted family member, friend, or professional to handle these personal affairs.

It is advisable to seek the expert advice of a lawyer in drawing up a will so that the decisions made about taxes, beneficiaries, and asset distribution will be legally binding. This process can relieve a person's family and friends of an enormous burden, particularly in cases of disputes or reservations about allocation of the testator's assets.

References

CHAPTER 1

AA (Alzheimer's Association). 2005. "Basics of Alzheimer's Disease: What It Is and What You Can Do." http://www.alz.org/national/documents/brochure_basicsofalz_low.pdf (accessed April 30, 2008).

Adelman, A. M., and M. P. Daly. 2005. "Initial Evaluation of the Patient with Suspected Dementia." *American Family Physician* 71, no. 9 (May 1).

Alagiakrishnan, K., and P. Blanchette. 2005. "Delirium." *eMedicine from WebMD*. July 28. http://www.emedicine.com/med/topic3006.htm (accessed September 2, 2006).

ASHP (American Society of Health-System Pharmacists). 2001. "New Study Reveals One-Third of Seniors Take Medications Prescribed by Two or More Physicians." Press release. August 6 http://www.ashp.org/s_ashp/sec_press_article.asp?CID=168&DID=2037&id=2528 (accessed September 2, 2006).

Barker, W. W., C. A. Luis, A. Kashuba, M. Luis, D. G. Harwood, D. Loewenstein, C. Waters, P. Jimison, E. Shepherd, S. Sevush, N. Graff-Radford, D. Newland, M. Todd, B. Miller, M. Gold, K. Heilman, L. Doty, I. Goodman, B. Robinson, G. Pearl, D. Dickson, and R. Duara. "Relative Frequencies of Alzheimer's Disease, Lewy Body, Vascular and Frontotemporal Dementia, and Hippocampal Sclerosis in the State of Florida

Brain Bank." 2002. *Alzheimer Disease and Associated Disorders* 16, no. 4 (October–December): 203–12.

Beers, M. H. 1997. "Explicit Criteria for Determining Potentially Inappropriate Medication Use by the Elderly: An Update." *Archives of Internal Medicine* 157: 1531–36.

Beers, M. H., J. G. Ouslander, I. Rollingher, D. B. Reuben, J. Brooks, and J. C. Beck. 1991. "Explicit Criteria for Determining Inappropriate Medication Use in Nursing Home Residents." *Archives of Internal Medicine* 151, no. 9: 1825–32.

Bottiglieri, T. 1996. "Folate, Vitamin B_{12} and Neuropsychiatric Disorders." *Nutrition Review* 54, no. 12 (December): 382–90.

Caird, F. I., and P. J. W. Scott. 1986. *Drug-Induced Disease in the Elderly: A Critical Survey of the Literature*. Drug-Induced Disorders series, vol. 2. Amsterdam: Elsevier Science.

Christensen, H. 2001. "What Cognitive Changes Can Be Expected with Normal Aging?" *Australian and New Zealand Journal of Psychiatry* 35 (December): 768.

Clarfield, A. M. 2003. "The Decreasing Prevalence of Reversible Dementias: An Updated Meta-analysis." *Archives of Internal Medicine* 163: 2219–29.

Correa-de-Araujo, R., E. G. Miller, and J. S. Banthin. 2005. "Gender Differences in Drug Use and Expenditures in a Privately Insured Population of Older Adults." *Journal of Women's Health* 14, no. 1: 73–81.

Crossley, K., and P. K. Peterson. 1998. "Infections in the Elderly—New Developments." *Current Clinical Topics in Infectious Diseases* 18: 75–100.

Derouesne, C., A. Alperovitch, N. Arvay, P. Migeon, F. Moulin, M. Vollant, J. R. Rapin, and M. Le Poncin. 1989. "Memory Complaints in the Elderly: A Study of 367 Community-Dwelling Individuals from 50–80 Years." *Archives of Gerontology and Geriatrics*, suppl. 1:151–63.

Dufour, M., and R. K. Fuller. 1995. "Alcohol in the Elderly." *Annual Review of Medicine* 46: 123–32.

Eastley, R., G. K. Wilcock, and R. S. Bucks. 2000. "Vitamin B_{12} Deficiency in Dementia and Cognitive Impairment: The Effects of Treatment on Neuropsychological Function." *International Journal of Geriatric Psychiatry* 15, no. 3 (May 18): 226–33. http://www.centre4activeliving.ca/publications/research_update/2006/dec06.html (accessed December 27, 2006).

Eriksson S. 1999. "Social and Environmental Contributants to Delirium in the Elderly." *Dementia and Geriatric Cognitive Disorders* 10: 350–52.

Espino, D. V., A. C. Jules-Bradley, C. L. Johnston, and C. P. Mouton. 1998. "Diagnostic Approach to the Confused Elderly Patient." *American Family Physician* 57, no. 6 (March 15).

Ewing, J. A. 1984. "Detecting Alcoholism: The CAGE Questionnaire." *Journal of the American Medical Association* 252: 1905–1907.

FDA (Food and Drug Administration). 2003. "Medications and Older People." *FDA Consumer Magazine.* Revised September 2003. Pub. no. FDA 03-1315C.

Fernandez, H. H., C. K. Wu, and B. R. Ott. 2003. "Pharmacotherapy of Dementia with Lewy Bodies." *Expert Opinion in Pharmacotherapy* 4, no. 11 (November): 2027–37.

Fick, D. M., J. W. Cooper, and E. Wade. 2003. "Updating the Beers Criteria for Potentially Inappropriate Medication Use in Older Adults: Results of a US Consensus Panel of Experts." *Archives of Internal Medicine* 163: 2716–24.

Fratiglioni, L., H. Wang, K. Ericsson, M. Maytan, and B. Winblad. 2000. "Influence of Social Network on Occurrence of Dementia: A Community-Based Longitudinal Study." *Lancet* 355: 1315–19.

Gale, C., C. Martyn, and C. Cooper. 1996. "Cognitive Impairment and Mortality in a Cohort of Elderly People." *British Medical Journal* 312: 608–11.

Gambert, S. A. 1997. "Is It Alzheimer's Disease?" *Postgraduate Medicine* 101, no. 6 (June). http://www.postgradmed.com/issues/1997/06_97/gambert.htm (accessed September 1, 2006).

Hutto, B. R. 1997. "Folate and Cobalamin in Psychiatric Illness." *Comprehensive Psychiatry* 6: 305–14.

IOM (Institute of Medicine). 1998. *Dietary Reference Intakes for Thiamin, Riboflavin, Niacin, Vitamin B6, Folate, Vitamin B12, Pantothenic Acid, Biotin and Choline.* Washington, DC: National Academy Press.

Kalaria, R. N. 2000. "Comparison between Alzheimer's Disease and Vascular Dementia: Implications for Treatment." *Neurological Research* 25, no. 6 (September): 661–64.

Kalaria, R. N., W. C. Low, A. E. Oakley, J. Y. Slade, P. G. Ince, C. M. Morris, and T. Mizuno. 2002. "CADASIL and Genetics of Cerebral Ischaemia." *Journal of Neural Transmission* 63: 75–90.

Kalimo, H., M. M. Ruchoux, M. Vitanen, R. N. Kalaruia. 2002. "CADASIL: A Common Form of Hereditary Arteriopathy Causing Brain Infarcts and Dementia." *Brain Pathology* 12, no. 3 (July): 371–84.

Khaira, J. S., and J. A. Franklyn. 1999. "Thyroid Conditions in Older Patients." *Practitioner* 243: 214–21.

Kivipelto, M. 2005. "Exercise in Midlife Could Reduce the Risk of Dementia and Alzheimer's Disease." *Lancet Neurology* (October 4). http://ki.se/ki/jsp/polopoly.jsp?d=933&a=3296&cid=940&l=en (accessed from Karolinska Institute, September 3, 2006).

Larson, E. B., W. A. Kukull, D. M. Buchner, and B. V. Reifler. 1987. "Adverse Drug Reactions Associated with Global Cognitive Impairment in Elderly Persons." *Annals of Internal Medicine* 107: 169–73.

Lesnik Oberstein, S. A., R. Van Den Boom, H. A. M. Middelkoop, M. D. Ferrari, Y. M. Knaap, H. C. Van Houwelingen, M. H. Breuning, M. A. Buchem, and J. Haan. 2003. "Incipient CADASIL." *Archives of Neurology* 60 (2003): 707–12.

McCue, J. D. 1999. "Treatment of Urinary Tract Infections in Long-Term Care Facilities: Advice, Guidelines and Algorithms." *Clinical Geriatrics*: 11–7.

McGlone, J., S. Gupta, D. Humphrey, S. Oppenheimer, T. Mirsen, and D. R. Evans. 1990. "Screening for Early Dementia Using Memory Complaints from Patients and Relatives." *Archives of Neurology* 47: 1189–93.

McQuinn, B. A., and D. H. O'Leary. 1987. "White Matter Lucencies on Computed Tomography, Subacute Arteriosclerotic Encephalopathy (Binswanger's Disease) and Blood Pressure." *Stroke* 18 (September/October): 900–905.

Mendez, M. F., A. Selwood, A. R. Mastry, and W. H. Frey. 1993. "Pick's Disease versus Alzheimer's Disease: A Comparison of Clinical Characteristics." *Neurology* 43: 289–92.

Mensah, G. A. 2004. "Special Focus: Heart Disease and Stroke." *Centers for Disease Control and Prevention, Chronic Disease News and Notes* 17, no. 1 (Fall).

Merck. 2006. *Merck Manual of Geriatrics*. "Dementia." February. http://www.merck.com/mrkshared/mmg/sec5/ch40/ch40e.jsp (accessed February 20, 2007).

Morrison, R. L., and I. R. Katz. 1989. "Drug-Related Cognitive Impairment: Current Progress and Recurrent Problems." *Annual Review of Gerontology and Geriatrics* 9: 232–79.

Neef, D., and A. Walling. 2006. "Dementia with Lewy Bodies: An Emerging Disease." *American Family Physician* 73, no. 7 (April 1).

Nielson, K. 2005. "Finding the Key to Successful Aging." *Neurobiology of Learning and Memory.* http://www.marquette.edu/research/aging.shtml (accessed September 1, 2006).

NINDS (National Institute of Neurological Disorders and Stroke). 2004. "The Dementias." NIH pub. no. 04-2252.

———. 2006. "Vasculitis Including Temporal Arteritis Information Page." January. http://www.ninds.nih.gov/disorders/vasculitis/vasculitis.htm (accessed September 1, 2006).

O'Connor, D., P. Pollitt, J. Hyde, C. P. Brook, B. B. Reiss, and M. Roth. 1988. "Do General Practitioners Miss Dementia in Elderly Patients?" *British Medical Journal* 297: 1107–10.

Olsen, C. G., and M. E. Clasen. 1998. "Senile Dementia of the Binswanger's Type." *American Academy of Family Physicians* (December). http://www.aafp.org/afp/981200ap/olsen.html (accessed September 1, 2006).

Oslin, D. 2000. "Prescription and Over-the-Counter Drug Misuse among the Elderly." *Geriatric Times* 1, no. 1 (May/June).

Pfefferbaum, A., E. V. Sullivan, D. H. Mathalon, and K. O. Lim. 1997. "Frontal Lobe Volume Loss Observed with Magnetic Resonance Imaging in Older Chronic Alcoholics." *Alcoholism: Clinical & Experimental Research* 21, no. 3: 521–29.

Rancourt, C., J. Moisan, L. Baillargeon, R. Verreault, D. Laurin, and J.-P. Grégoire. 2004. "Potentially Inappropriate Prescriptions for Older Patients in Long-Term Care." *BioMed Central Geriatrics* 4, no. 9.

Reid, J. 2005. "Polypharmacy; Causes and Effects in Older People." *Prescriber* (October 19). http://www.escriber.com/.../Images/Polypharmacy (accessed September 1, 2006).

Roman, G. C. 1987. "Senile Dementia of the Binswanger Type." *Journal of the American Medical Association* 258, no. 13 (October): 1782–88.

Roman, G. C., T. K. Tatemichi, T. Erkinjuntti, J. L. Cummings, J. C. Masdeu, J. H. Garcia, L. Amaducci, J.-M. Orgogozo, A. Brun, A. Hofman, D. M. Moody, M. D. O'Brien, T. Yamaguchi, J. Grafman, B. P. Drayer, D. A. Bennett, M. Fisher, J. Ogata, E. Kokmen, F. Bermejo, P. A. Wolf, P. B. Gorelick, K. L. Bick, A. K. Pajeau, M. A. Bell, C. DeCarli, A. Culebras, A. D. Korczyn, J. Bogousslavsky, A. Hartmann, and P. Scheinberg. 1993. "Vascular Dementia: Diagnostic Criteria for Research Studies.

Report of the NINDS-AIREN International Workshop." *Neurology* 43: 250–60.

Routledge, P. A., M. S. O'Mahony, and K. W. Woodhouse. 2004. "Adverse Drug Reactions in Elderly Patients." *British Journal of Clinical Pharmacology* 57: 121–26.

SAMSHA (Substance Abuse & Mental Health Services Administration). 1998. "Substance Abuse: Older Adults at Serious Risk." Press release. May 17. http://www.jointogether.org/news/research/pressreleases/1998/ substance-abuse-older-adults.html (accessed September 1, 2006).

Schmidt, M. L., V. Zhukreva, K. L. Newell, V. Lee, and J. Trojanowski. 2001. "Tau Isoform Profile and Phosphorylation State in Dementia Pugilistica Recapitulate Alzheimer's Disease." *Acta Neuropathologica* 101, no. 5 (May): 518–24.

Sharon, I., T. Erson, and R. Sharon. 2005. "Huntington Disease Dementia." *eMedicine from WebMD*. March 24. http://www.emedicine.com/med/ topic3111.htm (accessed September 1, 2006).

Thackery, E., ed. 2003. "Dementia." In *Gale Encyclopedia of Mental Disorders*. Farmington Hills, MI: Gale. http://health.enotes.com/mental-disorders-encyclopedia/dementia (accessed February 19, 2007).

Turnheim, K. 2003. "When Drug Therapy Gets Old: Pharmacokinetics and Pharmacodynamics in the Elderly." *Experimental Gerontology* 38: 843–53.

Valcour, V., K. Masaki, J. Curb, and P. Blanchette. 2000. "The Detection of Dementia in the Primary Care Setting." *Archives of Internal Medicine* 160: 2964–68.

Verrees, M., and W. Selman. 2004. "Management of Normal Pressure Hydrocephalus." *American Family Physician* 70, no. 6 (September 15). http://www.aafp.org/afp/20040915/1071.html (accessed September 3, 2006).

Volkow, N. D., G. J. Wang, J. E. Overall, R. Hitzemann, J. Fowler, N. Pappas, E. Frecska, and K. Piscani. 1997. "Regional Brain Metabolic Response to Lorazepam in Alcoholics during Early and Late Alcohol Detoxification." *Alcoholism: Clinical and Experimental Research* 21, no. 7: 1278–84.

Wilkinson, C., and H. Moskowitz. 2001. "Polypharmacy and Older Drivers: Literature Review." Unpublished manuscript. Southern California Research Institute, Los Angeles.

Williams, C. M. 2002. "Using Medications Appropriately in Older Adults." *American Family Physician* 66, no. 10 (November 15).

Wivel, M. E. 1988. "NIH Consensus Conference Stresses Need to Identify Reversible Causes of Dementia." *Hospital Community Psychiatry* 39: 22–23.

Zhanel, G. G., G. K. Harding, and D. R. Guay. 1990. "Asymptomatic Bacteriuria. Which Patients Should Be Treated?" *Archives of Internal Medicine* 150: 1389–96.

CHAPTER 2

AAGP (American Association for Geriatric Psychiatry). 2004. "Understanding the Most Common Dementing Disorder: Initiative on Alzheimer's Disease and Related Disorders." *American Association for Geriatric Psychiatry*. http://www.aagponline.org/p_c/alzheimers.asp (accessed September 11, 2006).

Adelman, A. M., and M. P. Daly. 2005. "Initial Evaluation of the Patient with Suspected Dementia." *American Family Physician* 71: 1745–50.

AGS (American Geriatrics Society). 2005. "Drug Treatment. Aging in the Know: Your Gateway to Aging and Resources on the Web." *American Geriatrics Society: Foundation for Health and Aging* (June 6). http://www.healthinaging.org/agingintheknow/chapters_ch_trial.asp?ch=6#changes (accessed August 30, 2006).

Barnes, D. E. 2003. "A Longitudinal Study of Cardiorespiratory Fitness and Cognitive Function in Healthy Older Adults." *Journal of the American Geriatrics Society* 51, no. 4 (April): 459–65.

Billups, S. J., D. C. Malone, and B. L. Carter. 2000. "Relationship between Drug Therapy Noncompliance and Patient Characteristics, Health-Related Quality of Life, and Health Care Costs." *Pharmacotherapy* 20, no. 8: 941–49.

Blalock, E. M., K.-C. Chen, K. Sharrow, J. P. Herman, N. M. Porter, T. C. Foster, and P. W. Landfield. 2003. "Gene Microarrays in Hippocampal Aging: Statistical Profiling Identifies Novel Processes Correlated with Cognitive Impairment." *Journal of Neuroscience* 23, no. 9 (May 1): 3807.

Bodarty, H., D. Pond, N. M. Kemp, G. Luscombe, L. Harding, K. Berman, and F. A. Huppert. 2000. "The GPCOG: A New Screening Test for Dementia Designed for General Practice." *Journal of the American Geriatric Society* 50, no. 3 (March): 530–34.

Botelho, R. J., and R. Dudrak. 1992. "Home Assessment of Adherence to Long-Term Medication in the Elderly." *Journal of Family Practice* 35: 61–65.

Boustani, M., C. M. Callahan, F. W. Unverzagt, M. G. Austrom, A. J. Perkins, B. A. Fultz, S. L. Hui, and H. C. Hendrie. 2005. "Implementing a Screening and Diagnosis Program for Dementia in Primary Care." *Journal of General Internal Medicine* 20, no. 7 (July): 572–77.

Boustani, M., B. Peterson, L. Hanson, R. Harris, and K. N. Lohr. 2003. "Screening for Dementia in Primary Care." *Annals of Internal Medicine* 138: 927–37.

Cohen, S., and T. B. Herbert. 1996. "Health Psychology: Psychological Factors and Physical Disease from the Perspective of Human Psychoneuroimmunology." *Annual Review of Psychology* 47: 113–42.

Conn, V. S. 1992. "Self-Management of Over-the-Counter Medications by Older Adults." *Public Health Nursing* 9, no. 1: 29–36.

Coons, S. J., S. L. Sheahan, S. S. Martin, J. Hendricks, C. A. Robbins, and J. A. Johnson. 1994. "Predictors of Medication Noncompliance in a Sample of Older Adults." *Clinical Therapeutics* 16: 110–17.

FDA (Food and Drug Administration). 2003. "Medications and Older People." September. Pub. no. FDA 03–1315C.

Folstein, M. F., S. E. Folstein, and P. R. McHugh. 1975. "Mini Mental Status Examination (MMSE)." *Journal of Psychiatric Research* 12: 189–98.

Ganguli, M., H. H. Dodge, C. Shen, and S. T. DeKosky. 2004. "Mild Cognitive Impairment, Amnestic Type: An Epidemiologic Study." *Neurology* 63, no. 1: 115–21.

Gazzaley, A. 2005. "Aging and Memory." *Nature Neuroscience* (October): 1298–1300.

Glisky, E. L., S. R. Rubin, and P. S. R. Davidson. "Source Memory in Older Adults: An Encoding or Retrieval Problem?" 2001. *Journal of Experimental Psychology: Learning, Memory, and Cognition* 27: 1131–46.

Gouras, G. K. 2001. "Current Theories for the Molecular and Cellular Pathogenesis of Alzheimer's Disease." *Cambridge Journals Online* (May 31). http://journals.cambridge.org/action/displayAbstract?fromPage=online &aid=168668# (accessed August 30, 2006).

Grace, J., and M. Amick. 2005. "Cognitive Screening of Older Adults." *Medicine and Health Rhode Island* 88, no. 1: 8–11.

Heinrich, J. "Health Products for Seniors: Potential Harm from 'Anti-Aging' Products." Statement before Special Committee on Aging, US Senate. http://www.gao.gov/new.items/d011139t.pdf (accessed May 6, 2008).

Jorm, A. F. 2000. "Is Depression a Risk Factor for Dementia or Cognitive Decline? A Review." *Gerontology* 46: 219–27.

Kane, R. L., J. G. Ouslander, and I. Abrass, eds. 1999. "Drug Therapy." In *Essentials of Clinical Geriatrics*, 4th ed., 379–411. New York: McGraw-Hill.

Lopez, O. L. 2003. "Risk Factors for Mild Cognitive Impairment in the Cardiovascular Health Study." *Archives of Neurology* 60 (October): 1394–99.

Lopez O. L., W. J. Jagust, S. T. DeKosky, J. T. Becker, A. Fitzpatrick, C. Dulberg, J. Breitner, C. Lyketsos, B. Jones, C. Kawas, M. Carlson, and L. H. Kuller. 2003. "Prevalence and Classification of Mild Cognitive Impairment in the Cardiovascular Health Study Cognition Study: Part 1." *Archives of Neurology* 60: 1385–89.

Lyketsos, C. G. 2005. "Population-Based Study of Medical Comorbidity in Early Dementia and Cognitive Impairment, No Dementia (CIND)." *American Journal of Geriatric Psychiatry* 13 (August): 656–64.

McKhann, G., and M. Albert. 2002. "Keep Your Brain Young." *Johns Hopkins Medical Newsletter: Health after 50*. August.

McKhann, G., D. Drachman, M. Folstein, R. Katzman, D. Price, and E. M. Stadlan. 1984. "Clinical Diagnosis of Alzheimer's Disease: Report of the NINCDS-ADRDA Work Group under the Auspices of the US Department of Health and Human Service's Task Force on Alzheimer's Disease." *Neurology* 34, no. 1 (July).

Merck. 2000. *Merck Manual of Geriatrics*. 3rd. ed. Edited by Mark H. Beers and Robert Berkow. New Jersey: Merck & Co.

Moore, A. R., and S. T. O'Keeffe. 1999. "Drug-Induced Cognitive Impairment in the Elderly." *Drugs & Aging* 15, no. 1 (July): 15–28.

Morris, J. C., and J. Cummings. 2005. "Mild Cognitive Impairment Represents Early-Stage Alzheimer's Disease." *Journal of Alzheimer's Disease* 7, no. 3: 235–39.

Newson, R. S., and E. B. Kemps. "Cardiorespiratory Fitness as a Predictor of Successful Cognitive Ageing." 2006. *Journal of Clinical and Experimental Neuropsychology* 28, no. 6 (August): 949–67.

NIA (National Institute on Aging). 2001. *Portfolio for Progress*. October.

————. 2004. "Donepezil May Have Short-Term Benefit for Mild Cognitive Impairment; More Analyses Needed to Assess Clinical Implications of New Data." 2004. *National Institute on Aging (NIA) News: AD Research Update*. July 18.

Patterson, C. J., and D. A. Gass. 2001. "Screening for Cognitive Impairment and Dementia in the Elderly." *Canadian Journal of Neurological Science* 28, suppl. 1 (February): S42–51.

Petersen, R. C., R. Doody, A. Kurz, R. C. Mohs, J. C. Morris, P. V. Rabins, K. Ritchie, M. Rossor, L. Thal, and B. Winblad. 2001. "Current Concepts in Mild Cognitive Impairment." *Archives of Neurology* 58, no. 12 (December): 1985–92.

Petersen, R. C., G. E. Smith, S. C. Waring, R. J. Ivnik, E. G. Tangalos, and E. Kokmen. 1999. "Mild Cognitive Impairment: Clinical Characterization and Outcome." *Archives of Neurology* 56, no. 3: 303–308.

Petersen, R. C., J. C. Stevens, M. Ganguli, E. G. Tangalos, J. L. Cummings, and S. T. DeKosky. 2001. "Practice Parameter: Early Detection of Dementia: Mild Cognitive Impairment (An Evidence-Based Review): Report of the Quality Standards Subcommittee of the American Academy of Neurology." *Neurology* 56: 1133–42.

Prichep, L. 2005. "A New Analysis of a Standard Brain Test May Help Predict Dementia." October 6. http://www.sciencedaily.com/releases/2005/10/051006084213.htm (accessed August 28, 2006).

Raji, M. A. 2005. "Ethnic Differences in Herb and Vitamin/Mineral Use in the Elderly." *Annals of Pharmacotherapy* 39 (June): 1019–23.

Rowe, J. W., and R. L. Kahn. 1997. "Successful Aging." *Gerontologist* 37: 433–40.

Stadtman, E. R. 1992. "Protein Oxidation and Aging." *Science* 257 (August 28): 1220–24.

Voit, S. 2002. "Insights on Maintaining Cognitive Health." *NIH Record* 54, no. 25 (December 10).

Wallman. 2004. Federal Interagency Forum on Aging Related Statistics, K. Wallman, chief statistician. Office of Management and Budget.

Williams, C. M. 2002. "Using Medications Appropriately in Older Adults." *American Family Physician* 66, no. 10 (November 15): 1917–24.

Zagaria, M. A. 2002. "Senior Health Maintenance." *US Pharmacist* (June): 35–38.

Zahn, C., I. Arispe, E. Kelley, T. Ding, C. W. Burt, J. Shinogle, and D. Stryer. 2005. "Ambulatory Care Visits for Treating Adverse Drug Effects in the United States, 1995–2001." *Journal on Quality and Patient Safety* 31, no. 7 (July): 372–78.

CHAPTER 3

AA (Alzheimer's Association). 2007. "Alzheimer's Disease Prevalence Rises." *Alzheimer News.* http://www.alz.org/news_and_events_rates _rise.asp (accessed March 22).

Bertram, L., M. Hiltunen, M. Parkinson, M. Ingelsson, C. Lange, K. Ramasamy, K. Mullin, R. Menon, A. J. Sampson, M. Y. Hsiao, K. J. Elliott, G. Velicelebi, T. Moscarillo, B. T. Hyman, S. L. Wagner, K. D. Becker, D. Blacker, and R. E. Tanzi. 2005. "Family-Based Association between Alzheimer's Disease and Variants in UBQLNI." *New England Journal of Medicine* 352: 884–94.

Bonte, F. J., T. S. Harris, C. A. Roney, and L. S. Hynan. 2004. "Differential Diagnosis between Alzheimer's and Frontotemporal Disease by the Posterior Cingulate Sign." *Journal of Nuclear Medicine* 45, no. 5 (May 5): 771–74.

Bren, L. 2003. "Alzheimer's: Searching for the Cure." *FDA Consumer Magazine,* July/August. Pub no. FDA 04-1318C rev.

Brookmeyer, R., S. Gray, and C. Kawas. 1998. "Projections of Alzheimer's Disease in the United States and the Public Health Impact of Delaying Disease Onset." *American Journal of Public Health* 88, no. 9: 1337–42.

CDC (Centers for Disease Control and Prevention). 2003. "National Vital Statistics Report, 2003."

———. 2006. "Health Information for Older Adults: Mental Health." http://www.cdc.gov/aging/info (accessed April 10, 2006).

Clarke, N. A., and P. T. Francis. 2005. "Cholinergic and Glutamatergic Drugs in Alzheimer's Disease Therapy." *Expert Review of Neurotherapeutics* 5, no. 5 (September): 671–82.

Colcombe, S. J., A. F. Kramer, K. I. Erickson, P. Scalf, E. McAuley, N. J. Cohen, A. Webb, G. J. Jerome, D. X. Marquez, and S. Elavsky. 2004. "Cardiovascular Fitness, Cortical Plasticity, and Aging." *Proceedings of the National Academy of Sciences, USA* 101, no. 9: 3316–21.

Dodge, H. H., and C. Shen. 2003. "Functional Transitions and Active Life Expectancy Associated with Alzheimer's Disease." *Archives of Neurology* 60: 253–59.

Doraiswamy, P. M., J. Leon, and J. L. Cummings. 2002. "Prevalence and Impact of Comorbidity in Alzheimer's Disease." *Journals of Gerontology Series A: Biological Sciences and Medical Sciences* 57: M173–77.

EPA (Environmental Protection Agency). 2006. "Aging and Toxic Response: Issues Relevant to Risk Assessment." Pub. no. EPA/600/P-03/004A. http://cfpub.epa.gov/ncea/cfm/recordisplay.cfm?deid=156648 (accessed May 9, 2008).

Ferri, C. P., M. Prince, C. Brayne, H. Brodaty, L. Fratiglioni, M. Ganguli, K. Hall, K. Hasegawa, H. Hendrie, Y. Huang, A. Jorm, C. Mathers, P. R. Menezes, E. Rimmer, M. Scazufca, and Alzheimer's Disease International. 2005. "Global Prevalence of Dementia: A Delphi Consensus Study." *Lancet* 366: 2112–17.

Folstein, M. F., S. E. Folstein, and P. R. McHugh. 1975. "Mini-Mental State: A Practical Method for Grading the State of Patients for the Clinician." *Journal of Psychiatric Research* 12: 189–98.

Friedman, S. M., D. M. Steinwachs, P. J. Rathouz, L. C. Burton, and D. B. Mukamel. 2005. "Characteristics Predicting Nursing Home Admission in the Program of All-Inclusive Care for Elderly People." *Gerontologist* 45: 157–66.

Graham, N. 2001. "World Health Report, 2001." http://www.who.int/multimedia/whr2001/audio.html (accessed August 26, 2006).

Hebert, L. E., P. A. Scherr, J. L. Bienias, D. A. Bennett, and D. A. Evans. 2003. "Alzheimer's Disease in the US Population: Prevalence Estimates Using the 2000 Census." *Archives of Neurology* 60, no. 8 (August): 1119–22.

Hoyert, D. L., and H. M. Rosenberg. 1999. "Mortality from Alzheimer's Disease: An Update." *National Vital Statistics Report* 47, no. 20 (June 30): 1–8.

Kepe, V. 2004. "Tracking Alzheimer's: UCLA Scientists Use FDDNP-PET to Detect and Quantify Alzheimer's Disease in Living Patients." *Society for Nuclear Medicine.* June 21. http://www.interactive.snm.org/index .cfm (accessed August 6, 2006).

Koppel, R. 2002. "Alzheimer's Disease: The Costs to US Businesses in

2002." US Chamber of Commerce, Long-Term Care Symposium, June 27. http://www.alz.org/national/documents/report_alzcosttobusiness.pdf (accessed May 8, 2008).

Korczyn, A. D. 2002. "Homocysteine, Stroke, and Dementia." *Stroke* 33: 2343.

Larson, E. B., M. F. Shadlen, L. Wang, W. C. McCormick, J. D. Bowen, L. Teri, and W. A. Kukull. 2004. "Survival after Initial Diagnosis of Alzheimer's." *Annals of Internal Medicine* 140, no. 7: 501–509.

Levey, A. 2001. "Do You Know What to Look for in Alzheimer's Patients?" *ACP-ASIM Observer*, June. http://www.acponline.org/journals/news/jun01/alzheimers (accessed August 28, 2006).

Lewin Group. 2004. "Saving Lives, Saving Money: Dividends for Americans Investing in Alzheimer Research." A Report from the Lewin Group, commissioned by the Alzheimer's Association. Washington, DC.

Lopez, O., J. Becker, S. Wisniewski, J. Saxton, D. Kaufer, and S. DeKoskyal. 2002. "Cholinesterase Inhibitor Treatment Alters the Natural History of Alzheimer's Disease." *Journal of Neurology, Neurosurgery and Psychiatry* 72, no. 3 (March): 310–14.

Luchsinger, J., M. X. Tang, and J. Miller. 2007. "Relation of Higher Folate Intake to Lower Risk of Alzheimer's Disease in the Elderly." *Archives of Neurology* 64: 86–92.

McIlroy, S. P., K. B. Dynan, J. T. Lawson, C. C. Patterson, and A. P. Passmore. 2002. "Moderate Elevations of Homocysteine Are Associated with a More Than Five-Fold Increase in the Risk for Stroke." *Stroke* (October 4).

Mehta, K. M., K. Yaffe, and K. E. Covinsky. 2002. "Cognitive Impairment, Depressive Symptoms, and Functional Decline in Older People." *Journal of the American Geriatrics Society* 50, no. 6 (June): 1045–50.

Miller, C. A. 2004. "Update on Dementia Medications for 2004." *Geriatric Nursing* 25, no. 1 (March 8): 56. http://www.medscape.com/viewarticle/470704 (accessed September 24, 2006).

Mosconi, L., A. Pupi, M. T. R. De Cristofaro, M. Fayyaz, S. Sorbi, and K. Herholz. 2004. "Functional Interactions of the Entorhinal Cortex: An 18F-FDG PET Study on Normal Aging and Alzheimer's Disease." *Journal of Nuclear Medicine* 45, no. 3: 382–92.

National Center for Health Statistics. 2005. "Leading Causes of Death in the US." *National Vital Statistics Reports*. March 7. http://www.statisticstop10.com/Causes_of_Death_in_US (accessed August 20, 2006).

NIA (National Institute on Aging), NIH (National Institutes of Health), and HHS (US Department of Health and Human Services). 2003. "Progress Report on Alzheimer's Disease, 2003." http://www.nia.nih.gov/NR/rdonlyres/0C3612EF-3C01-44EA-899B-223909A6DEEE/0/2003_Progress_Report_on_AD.pdf (accessed May 8, 2008).

NIH (National Institutes of Health). 2003. "Alzheimer's Disease Progress Report 2001." July. Pub. no. 03-5333.

———. 2005. "Genes, Lifestyles and Crossword Puzzles: Can Alzheimer's Disease Be Prevented?" May. Pub. no. 05-5503.

———. 2005. "Research Advances at NIH: Progress Report on Alzheimer's Disease, 2004–2005."

NIMH (National Institute of Mental Health). "The Numbers Count: Mental Disorders in America." http://www.nimh.nih.gov/health/publications/the-numbers-count-mental-disorders-in-america.shtml (accessed May 8, 2008).

NINDS (National Institute of Neurological Disorders and Stroke). 2004. "The Dementias." NIH pub. no. 04-2252.

Petersen, R. C., J. C. Stevens, M. Ganguli, E. G. Tangalos, J. L. Cummings, and S. T. DeKosky. 2001. "Practice Parameter: Early Detection of Dementia: Mild Cognitive Impairment (An Evidence-Based Review)." *Neurology* 56: 1133–42.

Provenzano, G., S. Duttagupta, T. McRae, V. Mastey, B. Ellis, and J. Ieni. 2001. "Delays in Nursing Home Placement for Patients with Alzheimer's Disease Associated with Treatment with Donepezil May Have Health Care Cost-Saving Implications." *Value in Health* 4, no. 2: 158.

Relkin, N. 2002. "Diagnosis of Alzheimer's Disease." Eighth International Conference on Alzheimer's Disease and Related Disorders. July 20–25.

Saxton, J., O. L. Lopez, and G. Ratcliff. 2004. "Preclinical Alzheimer's Disease: Neuropsychological Test Performance 1.5 to 8 Years Prior to Onset." *Neurology* 63, no. 12: 2341–47.

Seshdri, S., A. Beiser, J. Selhub, P. Jacques, I. Rosenberg, R. D'Agostino, P. Wilson, and P. Wolf. 2002. "Plasma Homocysteine as a Risk Factor for Dementia and Alzheimer's Disease." *New England Journal of Medicine* 346: 476–83.

Smith, G. E. "Early Onset Alzheimer's: An Interview with a Mayo Clinic Specialist." CNN.com. http://www.cnn.com/HEALTH/library/AZ/00009.html (accessed May 9, 2008).

Thompson, P. M., K. M. Hayashi, G. de Zubicaray, A. L. Janke, S. E. Rose, J. Semple, D. Herman, M. S. Hong, S. S. Dittmer, D. M. Doddrell, and A. W. Toga. 2003. "Dynamics of Gray Matter Loss in Alzheimer's Disease." *Journal of Neuroscience* 23, no. 3: 994–1005.

Truschke, E. *World Alzheimer Congress 2000.* http://www.seniorjournal .com/NEWS/2000%20Files/July%2000/FTR-07-20-00AlzConf.htm (accessed August 2, 2006).

Weaver, J. 2004. "Alzheimer's Anxiety: An Epidemic Looming, Americans Hope to Hang On to Their Memories." MSNBC. November 28. http:// www.msnbc.msn.com/id/6346873 (accessed August 25, 2006).

Wolfe, M. 2006. "Shutting Down Alzheimer's." *Scientific American* 294, no. 5: 60–67.

Wygaard, H. A., and G. Albreksten. 1992. "Risk Factors for Admission to a Nursing Home: A Study of Elderly People Receiving Home Nursing." *Scandinavian Journal of Primary Health Care* 10: 128–33.

CHAPTER 4

AAGP (American Association for Geriatric Psychiatry). 2001. "Late Life Depression." *Fact Sheet.*

———. N.d. "Depression in Late Life: Not a Natural Part of Aging." http://www.gmhfonline.org/gmhf/consumer/factsheets/depression_lateli fe.html (accessed May 9, 2008).

Abeloos, J., G. Rolly, J. Timperman, and A. Watson. 1985. "Anaesthetic and Medicolegal Problems in Patients Intoxicated by Alcohol." *Medicine, Science and the Law* 25: 131–35.

Atkinson, R. M., R. L. Tolson, and J. A. Turner. 1990. "Late versus Early Onset Problem Drinking in Older Men." *Alcoholism: Clinical and Experimental Research* 14, no. 4: 574–79.

Bartels, S. J., F. C. Blow, L. M. Brockmann, and A. D. Van Citters. 2005. "Substance Abuse and Mental Health among Older Americans: The State of the Knowledge and Future Directions." Report prepared for Older American Substance Abuse and Mental Health Technical Assistance Center/Substance Abuse and Mental Health Services. August 11. http://www.samhsa.gov/OlderAdultsTAC/SA_MH_%20AmongOlder Adultsfinal102105.pdf (accessed November 2, 2006).

Bucholz, K. K., V. M. Hesselbrock, J. J. Shayka, J. I. Nurnberger, M. A. Schuckit, I. Schmidt, and T. Reich. 1995. "Reliability of Individual Diagnostic Criterion Items for Psychoactive Substance Dependence and the Impact on Diagnosis." *Journal of Studies on Alcohol* 56: 500–505.

Browne, J. P., V. A. O'Doherty, and H. M. McGee. 1997. "General Practitioner and Public Health Nurse Views of Nutritional Risk Factors in the Elderly." *Irish Journal of Medicine and Science* 166, no. 1: 23–25.

Center for Substance Abuse Treatment. 1998. "Substance Abuse: Older Adults at Serious Risk." Press release. May 7. http://www.jointogether.org/news/research/pressreleases/1998/substance-abuse-older-adults.html (accessed August 24, 2006).

Chen, J. H., A. J. Bierhals, H. G. Prigerson, S. V. Kasl, C. M. Mazure, and S. Jacobs. 1999. "Gender Differences in the Effects of Bereavement-Related Psychological Distress in Health Outcomes." *Psychological Medicine* 29, no. 2: 367–80.

Conwell Y. 2001. "Suicide in Later Life: A Review and Recommendations for Prevention." *Suicide and Life Threatening Behavior* 31, suppl.: 32–47.

Conwell, Y., and D. Brent. 1995. "Suicide and Aging: Patterns of Psychiatric Diagnosis." *International Psychogeriatrics* 7, no. 2: 149–64.

Coupland, N., J. Coupland, and H. Giles. 1988. "Elderly Self-Disclosure: Interactional and Intergroup Issues." *Language and Communication* 8: 109–31.

Edwards, R. 1985. "Anaesthesia and Alcohol." *British Medical Journal* 291: 423–24.

FDA (Food and Drug Administration). 2003. *Federal Consumer Information Center* (September).

Fraser, A. G. 1997. "Pharmacokinetic Interactions between Alcohol and Other Drugs." *Clinical Pharmacokinetics* 33: 79–90.

Gallo, J. J., S. D. Ryan, and D. Ford. 1999. "Attitudes, Knowledge, and Behavior of Family Physicians regarding Depression in Late Life." *Archives of Family Medicine* 8, no. 3 (May/June): 249–56.

Gambert, S. R., and K. K. Katsoyannis. 1995. "Alcohol-Related Medical Disorders of Older Heavy Drinkers." In *Alcohol and Aging*, edited by Thomas Beresford and Edith Gomberg, 70–81. New York: Oxford University Press.

Harman, J. S., S. Crystal, and J. Walkup. 2003. "Trends in Elderly Patients'

Office Visits for the Treatment of Depression according to Physician Specialty: 1985–1999." *Springerlink* 30, no. 3 (July). www.springerlink .com/content/ax74k27413010w55 (accessed January 27, 2006).

Hasin, D., M. Weissman, and C. Mazure. 2005. "Depression Common among Baby Boomers." *Archives of General Psychiatry* (October).

HHS (US Department of Health and Human Services). 2007. "Health Information for Older Adults." http://www.cdc.gov/aging/info.htm (accessed June 3, 2008).

Husaini, B. A. 1997. "Predictors of Depression among the Elderly: Racial Differences over Time." *American Journal of Orthopsychiatry* 67, no. 1: 48–58.

Hylek, E. M., H. Heiman, and S. J. Skates. 1998. "Acetaminophen and Other Risk Factors for Excessive Warfarin Anticoagulation." *Journal of the American Medical Association* 279, no. 9 (March 4): 657–62.

James, R. T. 2005. "Clinical Practice Guidelines Give Little Guidance for Care of Older Patients." Editorial. *Archives of Internal Medicine* (August).

Jankowiak, J. 2002. "Depression May Be Another Risk for Alzheimer's Dementia: Your Doctor Can Help." *Neurology* 69: E4–E5 (accessed June 3, 2008).

Jeste, D. 2003. "Depression in Older Persons." *National Alliance on Mental Illness*. May.

Joseph, C. L. 1997. "Misuse of Alcohol and Drugs in the Nursing Home." In *Older Adults' Misuse of Alcohol, Medicines, and Other Drugs: Research and Practice Issues*, edited by Anne M. Gurnack, 228–54. New York: Springer.

Kurlowicz, L. H. 2003. "Depression." *GeroNurse Online*. http://www .geronurseonline.org/index.cfm?section_id=35&geriatric_topic_id=15 &sub_section_id=98&page_id=224&tab=2 (accessed September 24, 2006).

Kurlowicz, L. H., and NICHE Faculty. 1999. "Depression in Elderly Patients." In *Geriatric Nursing Protocols for Best Practice*, edited by I. Abraham, M. M. Bottrell, T. Fulmer, and M. D. Mezey, 111–30. New York: Springer.

Larsen, P. D., and J. L. Martin. 1999. "Polypharmacy and Elderly Patients." *Association of Operating Room Nurses Journal* 69, no. 3: 619–28.

Lebowitz, B. D., J. L. Pearson, and L. S. Schneider. 1997. "Diagnosis and

Treatment of Depression in Late Life. Consensus Statement Update." *Journal of the American Medical Association* 278, no. 14: 1186–90.

Leonard, R. 2006."Depression Triples the Likelihood That a Nursing Home Resident with Dementia Will Be Physically Aggressive." *Archives of Internal Medicine* (June 26).

Levine, N. 1997. "Pruritic Rash of the Hands and Feet." *Geriatrics* 52, no. 6: 29.

Liberto, J. G., D. W. Oslin, and P. E. Ruskin. 1992. "Alcoholism in Older Persons: A Review of the Literature." *Hospital and Community Psychiatry* 43: 975–84.

Little, J. T., C. F. Reynolds, M. A. Dew, E. Frank, A. Begley, M. Miller, C. Cornes, S. Mazumdar, J. Perel, and D. Kupfer. 1998. "How Common Is Resistance to Treatment in Recurrent, Nonpsychotic Geriatric Depression?" *American Journal of Psychiatry* 155, no. 8: 1035–38.

MacNair, T. 2006. "Depression in Elderly People." BBC Health. February 1. http://www.bbc.co.uk/health/conditions/depressionelderly1.shtml (accessed March 4, 2006).

Marom, E. M., H. P. McAdams, J. J. Erasmus, and P. C. Goodman. 1999. "The Many Faces of Pulmonary Aspiration." *American Journal of Roentgenolgy* 172: 121–28.

Merck. 1999. *Merck Manual of Diagnosis and Therapy.* 17th ed. Edited by Mark H. Beers and Robert Berkow. Whitehouse Station, NJ: Merck & Co.

———. 2000. *Merck Manual of Geriatrics.* 3rd ed. Chapter 33, "Depression." http://www.merck.com/mrkshared/mmg/sec4/ch33/ch33a.jsp (accessed February 23, 2007).

Michaelson, D., C. Stratakis, L. Hill, J. Reynolds, E. Galliven, G. Chrousos, and P. Gold. 1999. "Bone Mineral Density in Women with Depression." *New England Journal of Medicine* 335: 1176–80.

Miniño, A. M., E. Arias, and K. D. Kochanek. 2002. "Deaths: Final Data for 2000." *National Vital Statistics Reports* 50, no. 15.

Mor, V., C. A. McHorney, and S. Sherwood. 1986. "Secondary Morbidity among the Recently Bereaved." *American Journal of Psychiatry* 143: 158–63.

Morales, K., M. Wittink, C. Datto, S. DiFilippo, M. Cary, T. TenHave, and I. R. Katz. 2006. "Simvastatin Causes Changes in Affective Processes in Elderly Volunteers." *Journal of the American Geriatrics Society* 54: 70–76.

Moscicki, E. K. 2001."Epidemiology of Completed and Attempted Suicide: Toward a Framework for Prevention." *Clinical Neuroscience Research* 1: 310–23.

Neel, A. M. 1996. "Comorbid Disorders: Anxiety and Depression in the Nursing Home Resident." *Journal of the American Society of Consultant Pharmacists* 11, suppl. 4.

NIA (National Institute on Aging). 1999. "Diversity in Medication Use and Outcomes in Aging Populations." Pa. no. PA-99-097, May 7.

NIAAA (National Institute on Alcohol Abuse and Alcoholism). 1998. "Drinking in the United States: Main Findings from the 1992 National Longitudinal Alcohol Epidemiologic Survey (NLAES)." Pub. no. 99-3519.

NIH (National Institutes of Health). 1991. "Diagnosis and Treatment of Depression in Late Life." NIH Consensus Development Conference Statement, November 4–6. http://consensus.nih.gov/1991/1991 DepressionLateLife086html.htm (accessed May 9, 2008).

NIMH (National Institute of Mental Health). 2003. "Older Adults: Depression and Suicide Facts." Pub. no. 03-4593, revised May 2003. http://www.nimh.nih.gov/publicat/elderlydepsuicide.cfm (accessed March 23, 2005).

OSP (Office of Statistics and Programming), NCIPC (National Center for Injury Prevention and Control), and CDC (Centers for Disease Control and Prevention). "Web-Based Injury Statistics Query and Reporting System." (WISQARSTM) http://www.cdc.gov/ncipc/wisqars/default .htm (accessed April 2, 2005).

Peterson, M. G., J. P. Allegrante, A. Augurt, L. Robbins, C. R. Mackenzie, and C. N. Cornell. 2000. "Major Life Events as Antecedents to Hip Fracture." *Journal of Trauma-Injury Infection & Critical Care* 48, no. 6 (June): 1096–1100.

Pies, R., and D. Rogers. 2005. "The Recognition and Treatment of Depression: A Review for the Primary Care Clinician." *Medscape.* September 30. http://www.medscape.com/viewprogram/4572 (accessed March 10, 2006).

Prigerson, H. G., A. J. Bierhals, S. V. Kasl, C. F. Reynolds III, M. K. Shear, N. Day, L. C. Beery, J. T. Newsom, and S. Jacobs. 1997. "Traumatic Grief as a Risk Factor for Mental and Physical Morbidity." *American Journal of Psychiatry* 154: 616–23.

Reed S. 2007. "Older Adults and Prescription Drug Abuse: An Emerging Public Policy Issue." Paper presented at the annual meeting of the Midwest Political Science Association Online. April. www.allacademic .com/meta/p198758_index.html (accessed April 23, 2008).

Reynolds, C. F., E. Frank, J. M. Perel, S. D. Imber, C. Cornes, M. D. Miller, S. Mazumdar, P. R. Houck, M. A. Dew, J. A. Stack, B. G. Pollock, and D. J. Kupfer. 1999. "Nortriptyline and Interpersonal Psychotherapy as Maintenance Therapies for Recurrent Major Depression: A Randomized Controlled Trial in Patients Older Than 59 Years." *Journal of the American Medical Association* 281, no. 1: 39–45.

Ross, H. 2000. "Recognizing and Treating Depression in Older Adults: Closing the Gap, Growing Older." Office of Minority Health Resource Center, US Department of Health and Human Services. May.

Rupke, S., D. Blecke, and M. Renfrow. 2006. "Cognitive Therapy for Depression." *American Family Physician* 73, no. 1 (January 1). http:// www.aafp.org/afp/20060101/83.html (accessed March 10, 2006).

Schultz, S. 2005. "Mental Illness in Older Adults: Effective Treatments." Outreach Partnership Program 2005, annual meeting. April 1. http:// www.nimh.nih.gov/health/outreach/partnership-program/meetings/ 2005/mental-illness-in-older-adults-effective-treatments.shtml (accessed May 9, 2008).

SDCHIP (San Diego Community Health Improvement Partners). 2001. "Depression: The Invisible Culprit." San Diego Community Health Needs Assessment 2001. http://www.sdchip.org/work_teams/wt_na/wt _na_pdfs/F-depression%20edited.pdf (accessed March 8, 2006).

SG (Surgeon General). 1999. *Mental Health: A Report of the Surgeon General—Executive Summary.* Rockville, MD: US Department of Health and Human Services, Substance Abuse and Mental Health Services Administration, Center for Mental Health Services, National Institutes of Health, National Institute of Mental Health.

Smith, S. 1991. "What Is Stress?" *Stress Management Strategies.* Fact sheet HE-2089. Florida Cooperative Extension Service. November.

Stewart, W. F., J. A. Ricci, E. Chee, S. R. Hahn, and D. Morganstein. 2003. "Cost of Lost Productive Work Time among US Workers with Depression." *Journal of the American Medical Association* 289: 3135–44.

Van Exel, E., R. G. Westendorp, M. L. Stek, W. van Tilburg, A. T. F. Beekman, and A. J. M. de Craen. 2001. "Patients with Late-Onset

Depression Have Poor Cognitive Function at Old Age." *Journal of the American Geriatric Society* 49, no. 2: 245–63.

Zubenko, G. S. 2001. "Recurrent Major Depression Involves Significant Genetic, Environmental Impact on Family Members." *American Journal of Medical Genetics*. http://www.pslgroup.com/dg/205bda.htm (accessed April 4, 2007).

CHAPTER 5

AA (Alzheimer's Association). 2007. "Alzheimer's Disease Prevalence Rates Rise to More than Five Million in the United States." *Alzheimer News*. March 20. http://www.alz.org/news_and_events_rates_rise.asp (accessed March 22, 2007).

AoA (Administration on Aging). 2004. *Caregivers Handbook*. US Administration on Aging.

Bayer, A. H., and L. Harper. 2000. "Fixing to Stay: A National Survey on Housing and Home Modification Issues." AARP. May. http://www.aarp.org/research/reference/publicopinions/aresearch-import-783.html (accessed May 9, 2008).

Bond, J. T., C. Thompson, E. Galinsky, and D. Prottas. 2002. "Executive Summary, Highlights of the National Study of the Changing Workforce." Families and Work Institute, New York. http://www.familiesandwork.org/summary/nscw2002.pdf (accessed March 8, 2006).

Brodaty, H., and L. F. Low. 2003. "Aggression in the Elderly." *Journal of Clinical Psychiatry* 64, suppl. 4: 36–43.

Burke, J. R., and J. C. Morgenlander. 1999. "Managing Common Behavioral Problems in Dementia. How to Improve Quality of Life for Patients and Families." *Postgraduate Medicine Online* 106, no. 5 (October 15). http://www.postgradmed.com/issues/1999/10_15_99/morgenlander.shtml (accessed October 15, 1999).

Carrillo, M. 2005. Director, medical and scientific affairs, Alzheimer's Association, Chicago; C. Milner, chief executive officer, International Council on Aging, Vancouver, British Columbia. *Lancet*. December 17.

CDC (Centers for Disease Control and Prevention). 2000. "The Costs of Fall Injuries among Older Adults." January 27. http://www.cdc.gov/ncipc/factsheets/fallcost.htm (accessed May 9, 2008).

Covinsky, K. E., R. Newcomer, P. Fox, J. Wood, L. Sands, K. Dane, and K. Yaffe. 2003. "Patient and Caregiver Characteristics Associated with Depression in Caregivers of Patients with Dementia." *Journal of General Internal Medicine* 18, no. 12 (December): 1006–14.

FCA (Family Caregiver Alliance). 2006. "Support for Working Family Caregivers: Paid Leave Policies in California and Beyond." June. http://www .caregiver.org/caregiver/jsp/content_node.jsp?nodeid=1679 (accessed May 20, 2008).

GAO (General Accounting Office). 1994. "Long-Term Care: Diverse, Growing Population Includes Millions of Americans of All Ages." Report to Congressional requesters. GAO/HEHS 95-26. http://www.gao .gov/archive/1995/he95026.pdf (accessed March 8, 2006).

HHS (US Department of Health and Human Services). 2005. *Women's Health USA 2005.* US Department of Health and Human Services, Health Resources and Services Administration. Rockville, MD: US Department of Health and Human Services. http://mchb.hrsa.gov/whusa _05/pages/0303hcwc.htm (accessed May 10, 2008).

HRI (Human Resource Institute). 2000. "Measuring the Impact of Caregiving Responsibilities in the Labor Force: Employer Perspective." www.ncoa.org/Downloads/Employee%20Caregiver%20Presentation .ppt (accessed March 8, 2006).

IOM (Institute of Medicine). 2004. "Health Literacy: A Prescription to End Confusion." Report brief. April 8.

Jackson, M. 2005. "Pressures of Eldercare Often Exacerbated by a Lack of Support in the Workplace." April 10. http://www.bostonworks.boston .com/globe/balance/archives (accessed March 9, 2006).

Johnson, R. W., and J. M. Wiener. 2006. "A Profile of Frail Older Americans and Their Caregivers." March 1. http://www.urban.org/publications/ 311284.html (accessed May 9, 2008).

Livingston, G., K. Johnston, C. Katona, J. Paton, C. G. Lyketsos, and Old Age Task Force of the World Federation of Biological Psychiatry. 2005. "Systematic Review of Psychological Approaches to the Management of Neuropsychiatric Symptoms of Dementia." *American Journal of Psychiatry* 162, no. 11 (November): 1996–2021.

Lynn, J., and D. Adamson. 2003. "Living Well at the End of Life. Adapting Health Care to Serious Chronic Illness in Old Age." *RAND Health.* White paper, WP-137.

MMMI (MetLife Mature Market Institute). 1999. "The MetLife Juggling Act Study: Balancing Caregiving with Work and the Costs Involved." http://www.caregiving.org/data/jugglingstudy.pdf (accessed May 9, 2008).

———. 2006. *"Metlife Caregiving Cost Study: Productivity Losses to U.S. Business."* July. Introduction, p. 5.

National Council on the Aging. "The Quiet Problem at Work: Business and Community Solutions for Employers and Caregivers." http://www.ncoa.org/Downloads/Employee%20Caregiver%20Presentation.ppt (accessed May 9, 2008).

National Family Caregivers Association. 2000. "Random Sample Survey of Family Caregivers: Men Now Make Up 44% of the Caregiving Population." Unpublished. Summer. http://www.alsa.org/patient/facts.cfm (accessed April 2, 2006).

Neal, M., and D. Wagner. 2001. "Working Caregivers: Issues, Challenges and Opportunities for the Aging Network." Issue brief for National Family Caregiver Support Program, Washington, DC.

O'Brian, J., L. Shomphe, and J. Caro. 2000. "Behavioral and Psychological Symptoms in Dementia in Nursing Home Residents: The Economic Implications." *International Psychogeriatrics* 12: 51–57.

Raskind, M. A. 1999. "Evaluation and Management of Aggressive Behavior in the Elderly Demented Patient." *Journal of Clinical Psychiatry* 60, suppl. 15: 45–49.

Samarrai, F. 2002. "Getting Older and Better." *Inside UVA Online.* November 22–December 5. http://www.virginia.edu/insideuva/2002.31/williams_mark.html (accessed March 13, 2007).

Schulz, R., S. H. Belle, S. J. Czaja, K. A. McGinnis, A. Stevens, and E. Zhang. 2004. "Long-Term Care Placement of Dementia Patients and Caregiver Health and Well-Being." *Journal of the American Medical Association* 292 (August 25): 961–67.

Spector, W. 2000. "The Characteristics of Long-Term Care Users." Agency for Healthcare Research and Quality report. November 8.

Stewart, J. T. 1995. "Management of Behavior Problems in the Demented Patient." *American Family Physician* (December). http://www.findarticles.com/p/articles/mi_m3225/is_n8_v52/ai_17857196 (accessed March 11, 2007).

Tampi, R. 2004. "Studies Point Out Risk of Depression High among Care-

givers." *Healthlink*. March. http:www.ynhh.com/healthlink/mental
health/mentalhealth_3_04.html (accessed May 9, 2008).

Tennstedt, S. 1999. "Family Caregiving in an Aging Society." March 3.
http://www.aoa.gov/prof/research/famcare.pdf (accessed May 10, 2008).

Trubo, R. 2002. "Men Are Caregivers Too." *WebMD Feature.* October 14.
http://www.medicinet.com/script/main/art.asp? (accessed March 11,
2007).

Usita, P. M., S. S. Hall, and J. C. Davis. 2004. "Role Ambiguity in Family
Caregiving." *Journal of Applied Gerontology* 23, no. 1: 20–39.

Wagner, D. 2003. "Workplace Programs for Family Caregivers: Good Business and Good Practice." August. Family Caregiver Alliance/National
Center on Caregiving report. http://www.caregiver.org/caregiver/jsp/
content/pdfs/op_2003_workplace_programs.pdf (accessed March 30,
2007).

Yandrick, R. M. 2001. "Elder Care Grows Up." *HR Magazine* 46, no. 11
(November): 72–77.

Yeh, J., and S. Lo. 2004. "Living Alone: Social Support and Feeling Lonely
among the Elderly." *Social Behavior and Personality* 32, no. 1: 129–38.

Young, L. 2002. "Women and Aging: Bearing the Burden of Long-Term
Care." Testimony at a joint hearing before the Special Committee on
Aging and the Subcommittee on Aging. Health, Education, Labor and
Pensions Committee of the US Senate. February 6.

CHAPTER 6

AAFP (American Academy of Family Physicians). 2006. "Homocysteine."
April. http://www.familydoctor.org/249.xml (accessed October 29,
2006).

AAGP (American Association for Geriatric Psychiatry). 2004. "Health Care
Professionals: Geriatrics and Mental Health—The Facts." http://www
.aagpgpa.org/prof/facts_mh.asp (accessed September 9, 2006).

ADA (American Dietetic Association). 2000. "Nutrition, Aging, and the
Continuum of Care." *Journal of the American Dietetic Association* 100,
no. 5 (May): 580–95.

ADEAR (Alzheimer's Disease Education and Referral Center). 2006. "The
Changing Brain in Alzheimer's Disease." August 29. http://www.nia

.nih.gov/Alzheimers/Publications/UnravelingTheMystery/Part1/Changing BrainInAlzheimer.htm (accessed October 10, 2006).

Andel, R., T. Hughes, and M. Crowe. 2005. "Strategies to Reduce the Risk of Cognitive Decline and Dementia." *AgingHealth* 1, no. 1 (August 1): 107–16.

Balaraman, R., and J. Shingala. 2002. "Molecule of the Millennium." *Indian Journal of Pharmacology* 34: 439–40. http://www.ncbi.nlm.nih.gov/ entrez/query.fcgi?cmd=Retrieve&db=PubMed&list_uids=10927860 &dopt=Abstract (accessed May 3, 2006).

Bennett, D. A., J. A. Schneider, J. L. Bienias, D. A. Evans, and R. S. Wilson. 2005. "Mild Cognitive Impairment Is Related to Alzheimer Disease Pathology and Cerebral Infarctions." *Neurology* 64, no. 5 (March 8): 834–41.

Benton, D., and P. Y. Parker. 1998. "Breakfast, Blood Glucose, and Cognition." *American Journal of Clinical Nutrition* 67: 772S–78S.

Blasko, D. 2005. "Why Do We Forget?" *Research Penn State*. August 15. http://www.rps.psu.edu/probing/forget.html (accessed October 3, 2006).

Blasko, D. G., and M. D. Hall. 1998. "Influence of Prosodic Boundaries on Comprehension of Spoken English Sentences." *Perception and Motor Skills* 87, no. 1 (August): 3–18.

Brown, A. S. 1991. "A Review of the Tip-of-the-Tongue Experience." *Psychological Bulletin* 109, no. 2 (March): 204–23. http://www.ncbi.nlm .nih.gov/entrez/query.fcgi?cmd=Retrieve&db=PubMed&list_uids =2034750&dopt=Abstract (accessed October 4, 2006).

Brunson, K., M. Eghbal-Ahmadi, R. Bender, and Y. Chen. 2001. "Brain Hormone May Hold Key to Memory Loss, Impaired Cognition, Caused by Unusual Stress during Infancy." News release. UCI Medical Center, University of California, Irvine. July 9. http://www.ucihealth.com/News/ Releases/BrainHormone.htm (accessed September 22, 2006).

Caballero, J., and M. Nahata. 2004. "Do Statins Slow Down Alzheimer's Disease? A Review." *Journal of Clinical Pharmacy and Therapeutics* 29, no. 3: 209–13.

Caprini, S., D. de Ronchi, A. R. Atti, M. Ujkaj, M. Morri, E. Dalmonte, A. Karp, and L. Fratiglioni. 2006. "Mental Activity and Dementia Risk." *Alzheimer's & Dementia* 2, no. 3 suppl. 1: S566 (abstract P4-170).

CDC (Centers for Disease Control and Prevention). 2006. "Healthy Aging, Preventing Disease and Improving Quality of Life among Older Americans."

Clarke, R. 2006. "Vitamin B12, Folate and the Prevention of Dementia." *New England Journal of Medicine* 354 (June 29): 2817–19.

Clarkson, T. W. 2003. "The Toxicology of Mercury: Current Exposures and Clinical Manifestations." *New England Journal of Medicine* 349, no. 18 (October 30): 1731–37.

Cohen, R. A., S. Grieve, K. Hoth, R. A. Paul, L. Sweet, D. Tate, J. Gunstad, L. Stroud, J. McCaffrey, B. Hitsman, R. Niaura, R. Clark, A. MacFarlane, R. A. Bryant, E. Gordon, and L. M. Williams. 2006. "Early Life Stress and Morphometry of the Adult Anterior Cingulate Cortex and Caudate Nuclei." *Biological Psychiatry* 59, no. 10 (May 15): 975–82.

Cowan, N. 2001. "The Magical Number 4 in Short-Term Memory: A Reconsideration of Mental Storage Capacity." *Behavioral and Brain Sciences* 24: 87–185.

Craft, S., J. Newcomer, S. Kanne, S. Dagogo-Jack, P. Cryer, Y. Sheline, J. Luby, A. Dagogo-Jack, and A. Alderson. 1996. "Memory Improvement Following Induced Hyperinsulinemia in Alzheimer's Disease." *Neurobiology of Aging* 17: 123–30.

Dark-Freudeman, A., R. L. West, and K. M. Viverito. "Future Selves and Aging: Older Adults' Memory Fears." *Educational Gerontology* 36, no. 2 (February 2006): 85–109.

Deschamps, V., P. Barberger-Gateau, E. Peuchant, and J. M. Orgogozo. 2001. "Nutritional Factors in Cerebral Aging and Dementia: Epidemiological Arguments for a Role of Oxidative Stress." *Neuroepidemiology* 20, no. 1 (February): 7–15.

Elias, M., L. Sullivan, R. D'Agostino, P. Elias, P. Jacques, J. Selhub, S. Seshadri, R. Au, A. Beiser, and P. Wolf. 2005. "Homocysteine and Cognitive Performance in the Framingham Offspring Study: Age Is Important." *American Journal of Epidemiology* 162, no. 7 (October 1).

Engelhart, M. J., M. I. Geerlings, A. Ruitenberg, J. C. Van Swieten, A. Hofman, J. C. Witteman, and M. M. Breteler. 2003. "Diet and the Risk of Dementia: Does Fat Matter? The Rotterdam Study." *Neurology* 60, no. 12 (June 24): 2020–21.

English, T. 2006. "Aging Well: Eating Right Is Worth the Effort." *Facts of Life: Issue Briefings for Health Reporters* 11, no. 7 (July).

Friedland, R. P., T. Fritsch, K. A. Smyth, E. Koss, A. J. Lerner, C. H. Chen, G. J. Petot, and S. M. Debanne. 2001. "Patients with Alzheimer's Disease Have Reduced Activities in Midlife Compared with Healthy Control-Group Members." *Proceedings of the National Academy of Sciences of the USA* 98: 3440–45.

Gatz, M. 2005. "Educating the Brain to Avoid Dementia: Can Mental Exercise Prevent Alzheimer's Disease?" *Public Library of Science, Medicine* 2, no. 1 (January). http://www.medicine.plosjournals.org (accessed September 21, 2006).

Giurgea, C. E. 1973. "The Nootropic Approach to the Pharmacology of the Integrative Activity of the Brain." *Conditional Reflex* 8: 108–15.

Goodwin, J. S., J. M. Goodwin, and P. J. Garry. 1983. "Association between Nutritional Status and Cognitive Functioning in a Healthy Elderly Population." *Journal of the American Medical Association* 249: 2917–21.

Griffin, K. 2005. "You're Wiser Now: A New Look at the Surprising Resilience and Growth Potential of the Human Brain." AARP. October. http://www.aarpmagazine.org/health/youre_wiser_now.html (accessed October 1, 2006).

Hall, C. B., J. Verghese, C. A. Derby, M. Katz, H. Buschke, G. Kuslansky, and R. Lipton. 2006. "Higher Educational and Occupational Achievement Are Associated with More Rapid Memory Decline in Preclinical Alzheimer's Disease: Evidence for Cognitive Reserve." *Alzheimer's & Dementia* 2, no. 3, suppl. 1: S19.

Helmuth, L. 1999. "Neural Teamwork May Compensate for Aging." *Science News*. April.

Hitti, M. 2006. "Diet, Exercise May Fend Off Dementia." WebMD. July 18. http://www.webmd.com/alzheimers/news/20060718/diet-exercise-dementia (accessed May 12, 2008).

Jick, H., G. L. Zornberg, S. S. Jick, S. Seshadri, and D. A. Drachman. 2000. "Statins and the Risk of Dementia." *Lancet* 356: 1627–31.

Juan, D., D. H. Zhou, J. Li, J. Y. Wang, C. Gao, and M. Chen. 2004. "A 2-Year Follow-Up Study of Cigarette Smoking and Risk of Dementia." *European Journal of Neurology* 11, no. 4 (April): 277–82.

Kalmijn, S., L. J. Launer, A. Ott, J. C. Witteman, A. Hofman, and M. M. Breteler. 1997. "Dietary Fat Intake and the Risk of Incident Dementia in the Rotterdam Study." *Annals of Neurology* 42: 776–82.

Kesler, S. R., H. F. Adams, C. M. Blasey, and E. D. Bigler. 2003. "Premorbid Intellectual Functioning, Education, and Brain Size in Traumatic Brain Injury: An Investigation of the Cognitive Reserve Hypothesis." *Applied Neuropsychology* 10: 153–62.

King, D. S., A. J. Wilburn, M. R. Wofford, T. K. Harrell, B. J. Lindley, and D. W. Jones. 2003. "Cognitive Impairment Associated with Atorvastatin and Simvastatin." *Pharmacotherapy* 23, no. 12 (December): 1663–67.

Kivipelto, M., T. Ngandu, T. Laatikainen, B. Winblad, H. Soininen, and J. Tuomilehto. 2006. "Risk Score for the Prediction of Dementia Risk in 20 Years among Middle-Aged People: A Longitudinal, Population-Based Study." *Lancet Neurology* 5, no. 9 (September): 735–41.

Kotulak, R. 1997. *Inside the Brain: Revolutionary Discoveries of How the Mind Works.* Kansas City, MO: Anreas and McMeely.

Koudinov, A. R., and N. V. Koudinova. 2001. "Brain Cholesterol Pathology Is the Cause of Alzheimer's Disease." *Therapeutics.* June. http://www.clinmed.netprints.org/cgi/content/full/2001100005v1 (accessed November 29, 2006).

Kuhn, H. G., T. D. Palmer, and E. Fuchs. 2001. "Adult Neurogenesis: A Compensatory Mechanism for Neuronal Damage." *European Archives of Psychiatry and Clinical Neuroscience* 251, no. 4 (August): 152–58.

Laitinen, M. H., E.-L. Helkala, U. Uusitalo, T. Ngandu, S. Rovio, M. Viitanen, A. Nissinen, J. Tuomilehto, H. Soininen, and M. Kivipelto. 2004. "Midlife Dietary Fats and the Risk of Late-Life Dementia: A Population-Based Study." *Neurobiology of Aging* 25: 399.

Lothian, K., and I. Philp. 2001. "Care of Older People: Maintaining the Dignity and Autonomy of Older People in the Healthcare Setting." *British Medical Journal* 322 (March 17): 668–70.

Mattson, M. P. 2000. "Existing Data Suggest That Alzheimer's Disease Is Preventable." *Annals of the New York Academy of Sciences* 924: 153–59.

McFarlane, A. 2005. "The Impact of Early Life Stress on Psychophysiological Personality and Behavioral Measures in 740 Non-clinical Subjects." *Journal of Integrative Neuroscience* 4, no. 1 (March): 27–40. http://www.ncbi.nlm.nih.gov/pubmed/16035139 (accessed May 12, 2008).

McMahon, J., T. J. Green, C. M. Skeaff, R. G. Knight, J. I. Mann, and S. M. Williams. 2006. "A Controlled Trial of Homocysteine Lowering and Cognitive Performance." *New England Journal of Medicine* 354, no. 26 (June 29): 2764–72.

Miller, G. 1956. "The Magical Number Seven, Plus or Minus Two: Some Limits on Our Capacity for Processing Information." *Psychological Review* 63, no. 2 (March): 81–97.

Miller, K. 2001. "Cholesterol—Don't Think without It: Heart Clogger Helps

Neurons Connect." *Science's SAGE KE*. November 14. http://www
.sageke.sciencemag.org/cgi/content/abstract/sageke;2001/7/nw26
(accessed September 27, 2006).

Mitka, M. "Aging Patients Are Advised 'Stay Active to Stay Alert.'" *Journal of the American Medical Association* 285: 2437–38.

Morley, J. E. 1997. "Anorexia of Aging: Physiologic and Pathologic." *American Journal of Clinical Nutrition* 66 (1997): 760–73.

———. 2000. "Diabetes Mellitus: A Major Disease of Older Persons." *Journal of Gerontology* 55: M255–56.

———. 2001. "Food for Thought." *American Journal of Clinical Nutrition* 74, no. 5 (November): 567–68.

Morris, M. 2006. "Good Fat, Bad Fat: The Facts about Omega-3." *Archives of Neurology* 63 (November): 1527–28.

NIA (National Institute on Aging). 2002. "Health Quackery: Spotting Health Scams." *Age Page*. September.

———. 2006. "Can Alzheimer's Disease Be Prevented?" *National Institute on Aging/Alzheimer's Disease Education and Referral Center*. http:// www.nia.nih.gov/Alzheimers/Publications/ADPrevented/chap01.htm (accessed September 24, 2006).

NIH (National Institutes of Health). 2001. Cognitive and Emotional Health: The Healthy Brain Workshop. National Institute Neurological Disorders and Stroke (NINDS), National Institute of Mental Health (NIMH), and National Institute of Aging (NIA). July 9–10.

———. 2006. "Genes, Lifestyles, and Crossword Puzzles: Can Alzheimer's Disease Be Prevented?" Pub. no. 06-5503. June.

Nussbaum, P. 2005. "Ten Tips for Maintaining Brain Health." *MetLife Mature Market Institute*. November. http://www.findarticles.com/p/ articles/mi_m0EIN/is_2005_Nov_16/ai n15800027 (accessed September 16, 2006)

OASIS. 2004. "Feed Your Brain." http://www.oasisnet.org/learn/h_brain.htm (accessed April 6, 2006).

Ott, A., A. J. Slooter, and A. Hofman. 1998. "Smoking and Risk of Dementia and Alzheimer's Based Cohort Study: The Rotterdam Study." *Lancet* 351 (June 30): 1840–43.

Passmore, P., R. Bullock, B. McGuinness, and S. Todd. 2006. "Blood Pressure Lowering in Patients without Prior Cerebrovascular Disease for Prevention of Cognitive Impairment and Dementia." *Hypertension News* 4.

Ranpura, A. 2000. "How We Remember and Why We Forget." *Brain Con-nection*. June. http://www.brainconnection.com/topics/?main=fa/ memory-formation (accessed October 1, 2006).

Rea, T., J. C. Breitner, and B. M. Psaty. 2005. "Statin Use and the Risk of Incident Dementia: The Cardiovascular Health Study." *Archives of Neurology* 62, no. 7 (July): 753–57.

Saxe, S., M. Wekstein, R. Kryscio, R. Henry, C. Cornett, D. Snowdon, F. Grant, F. Schmitt, S. Donegan, D. Wekstein, W. Ehmann, and W. Markesbery. 1999. "Alzheimer's Disease, Dental Amalgam, and Mercury." *Journal of the American Dental Association* 130, no. 2 (February): 191–99.

Scarmeas, N., G. Levy, M.-X. Tang, J. Manly, and Y. Stern. 2001. "Influence of Leisure Activity on the Incidence of Alzheimer's Disease." *Neurology* 57: 2236–42.

Scarmeas, N., and Y. Stern. 2003. "Cognitive Reserve and Lifestyle." *Journal of Clinical and Experimental Neuropsychology* 25, no. 5: 625–33.

Schaefer, E. 2006. "Good Fat, Bad Fat: The Facts about Omega-3." *Archives of Neurology* 63 (November): 1545–50.

Schaie, K. W. 2005. *Developmental Influences on Adult Intellectual Development: The Seattle Longitudinal Study.* New York: Oxford University Press.

Scott, H. D., and K. Laake. 2006. "Statins for the Prevention of Alzheimer's Disease." *Cochrane Library* 3.

SG (Surgeon General). 1999."Mental Health: A Report of the Surgeon General—Executive Summary." Rockville, MD. US Department of Health and Human Services, Substance Abuse and Mental Health Services Administration, Center for Mental Health Services, National Institutes of Health, National Institute of Mental Health, 1999.

Small, G. W. 2002. "What We Need to Know about Age-Related Memory Loss." *British Medical Journal* 324: 1502–1505.

Smith, A. P., R. Clark, and J. Gallagher. 1999. "Breakfast Cereal and Caffeinated Coffee: Effects on Working Memory, Attention, Mood and Cardiovascular Functioning." *Physiology & Behaviour* 1: 9–17.

Solfrizzi, V., F. Panza, F. Torres, F. Mastroianni, A. Del Parigi, A. Venezia, and A. Capurso. 1999. "High Monounsaturated Fatty Acids Intake Protects against Age-Related Cognitive Decline." *Neurology* 52: 1563–69.

Springer, M. V., A. R. McIntosh, G. Winocur, and C. L. Grady. 2005. "The Relation between Brain Activity during Memory Tasks and Years of Education in Younger and Older Adults." *Neuropsychology and Aging* 19, no. 2 (March): 181–92.

Staff, R. T., A. D. Murray, I. J. Deary, and L. J. Whalley. 2004. "What Provides Cerebral Reserve?" *Brain* 127, no. 5 (2004): 1191–99.

Stern, Y. 2002. "What Is Cognitive Reserve? Theory and Research Application of the Reserve Concept." *Journal of the International Neuropsychological Society* 8, no. 3 (March): 448–60.

———. 2004. "Complex Brain Circuits May Protect against Alzheimer's." *In Vivo* 3, no. 12 (November/December). http://www.cumc.columbia .edu/news/in-vivo/Vol3_Iss11_nov_dec_04/index.html (accessed September 19, 2006).

Stern, Y., C. Habeck, J. Moeller, N. Scarmeas, K. E. Anderson, H. J. Hilton, J. Flynn, H. Sackeim, and R. van Heertum. 2005. "Brain Networks Associated with Cognitive Reserve in Healthy Young and Old Adults." *Cerebral Cortex* 15: 394–402.

Travis, J. 2001. "Cholesterol Enables Nerve Cells to Connect." *Science News* 160, no. 20 (November 17). http://www.sciencenews.org/articles/ 20011117/fob3.asp (accessed September 27, 2006).

Tufts Health & Nutrition Letter. 2005. "Getting Smart about Alzheimer's: Scientists Find Clues in What We Eat, How Much Exercise We Get and What Medicines We Take." May. http://www.healthletter.tufts.edu/ issues/2005-05/alzheimers.html (accessed May 13, 2008).

Valenzuela, M., and P. Sachdev. 2006. "Brain Reserve: The Impact of Complex Mental Activity on Dementia Incidence, Cognitive Decline and Hippocampal Structure and Function." *Alzheimer's & Dementia* 2, no. 3, suppl, 1: S1676–8.

Vockell, E. L. 2006. "Forgetting." http://www.education.calumet.purdue .edu/vockell/EdPsyBook/Edpsy6/edpsy6_forgetting.htm (accessed October 9, 2006).

Waugh, N. C., and D. A. Norman. 1965. "Primary Memory." *Psychological Review* 72, no. 2: 89–104.

Whalley, L. J., I. J. Deary, C. L. Appleton, and J. M. Starr. 2004. "Cognitive Reserve and the Neurobiology of Aging." *Ageing Research Reviews* (November): 369–82.

Willis, S. L. 1990. "Current Issues in Cognitive Training Research." In *Aging* and Cognition: Mental Processes, Self-Awareness and Interventions, edited by Eugene A. Lovelace, 263–80. Amsterdam: North-Holland Press.

Woodward, M., H. Brodaty, M. Budge, G. Byrne, L. Flicker, J. Hecker, and S. Velandai. 2005. "Dementia: Can It Be Prevented?" Alzheimer's Australia Position Paper Number 6. August. http://www.alzheimers.org.au/ upload/dementiapreventedsept05.pdf (accessed September 19, 2006).

Zandi, P., L. Sparks, A. Kachaturian, J. Tschanz, M. Norton, M. Steinberg, K. A. Welsh-Bohmer, J. C. Breitner, and Cache County Study Investigators. 2005. "Do Statins Reduce Risk of Incident Dementia and Alzheimer Disease?" *Archives of General Psychiatry* 62, no. 2: 217–24.

CHAPTER 7

Adams, W. L., K. Barry, and M. Fleming. 1996. "Screenings for Problem Drinking in Older Primary Care Patients." *Journal of the American Medical Association* 276: 1964–67.

AGS (American Geriatrics Society) 2001. "Guideline for the Prevention of Falls in Older Persons." *Journal of the American Geriatrics Society* 49, no. 5 (May): 664–72.

Alexander, N. 2005. "Gait Disorders: Search for Multiple Causes." *Cleveland Clinic Journal of Medicine* 72, no. 7 (July 2005): 586. http://www .ccjm.org/PDFFILES/Alexander7_05.pdf (accessed May 13, 2008).

Alexander, N. B. 1999. "Gait Disorders in Older Adults." *Clinical Geriatrics* 7, no. 3 (March): 1070–1389. http://www.clinicalgeriatrics.com/article/ 1231 (accessed January 27, 2007).

AP (Associated Press). 2006. "Elderly Dying from Falls More Often." November 16. http://www.msnbc.msn.com/id/15753689 (accessed January 7, 2007).

Bakarich, A., V. McMillan, and R. Prosser. 1997. "The Effect of a Nursing Intervention on the Incidence of Older Patient Falls." *Australian Journal of Advanced Nursing* 15, no. 1 (September/November): 26–31.

Bell, A. J., J. K. Talbot-Stern, and A. Hennessy. 2000. "Characteristics and Outcomes of Older Patients Presenting to the Emergency Department after a Fall: A Retrospective Analysis." *Medical Journal of Australia* 173, no. 4: 176–77.

Bergland, A., G. B. Jarnlo, and K. Laake. 2003. "Predictors of Falls in the Elderly by Location." *Aging: Clinical and Experimental Research* 15: 43–50.

Bergland, A., A. M. Pettersen, and K. Laake. 1998. "Falls Reported among Elderly Norwegians Living at Home." *Physiotherapy Research International* 3: 164–74.

Billups, S. J., D. C. Malone, and B. L. Carter. 2000. "Relationship between Drug Therapy Noncompliance and Patient Characteristics: Health-Related Quality of Life and Health Care Costs." *Pharmacotherapy* 20, no. 8: 941–49.

Brown, J. S., E. Vittinghoff, J. F. Wyman, K. L. Stone, M. C. Nevitt, K. E. Ensrud, and D. Grady. 2001. "Urinary Incontinence: Does It Increase Risk for Falls and Fractures?" *Journal of the American Geriatrics Society* 49, no. 3 (March): 336–37.

Brunner, L. C., L. Eshilian-Oates, and T. Y. Kuo. 2003. "Hip Fractures in Adults/Radiologic Decision-Making." *American Family Physician* (February 1). http://www.aafp.org/afp/20030201/537.html (accessed December 27, 2006).

Butler, R. N., R. Davis, C. B. Lewis, M. E. Nelson, and E. Strauss. 1998. "Physical Fitness: Benefits of Exercise for the Older Patient." *Geriatrics* 53, no. 10: 46–62.

Callahan, C. M., and W. M. Tierney. 1995. "Health Services Use and Mortality among Older Primary Care Patients with Alcoholism." *Journal of the American Geriatrics Society* 43, no. 12 (December): 1378–83.

CDC (Centers for Disease Control and Prevention). 2001. "Unintentional Injury Prevention Program." *Activity Report, 2001.* http://www.cdc .gov/ncipc/pub-res/unintentional_activity/07_state_programs.htm (accessed February 7, 2007).

———. 2002. *Injury Fact Book.* http://www.cdc.gov/ncipc/factbook/15 _Falls_Among_Older_Adults.htm (accessed January 9, 2007).

———. 2007. "Fall Prevention Activities." http://www.cdc.gov/ncipc/ duip/FallsPreventionActivity.htm (accessed March 22, 2007).

———. 2005. Web-based Injury Statistics Query and Reporting System (WISQARS). http://www.cdc.gov/ncipc/wisqars (accessed December 15, 2006).

Chang, J. T., S. C. Morton, L. Z. Rubenstein, W. A. Mojica, M. Maglione, M. J. Suttorp, E. A. Roth, and P. G. Shekelle. 2004. "Interventions for the

Prevention of Falls in Older Adults: Systematic Review and Meta-analysis of Randomized Clinical Trials." *British Medical Journal* 328: 680.

Cooper, J. W. 1997. "Reducing Falls among Patients in Nursing Homes." *Journal of the American Medical Association* 278: 1742–43.

Cumming, R. G., M. Thomas, G. Szonyi, G. Salkeld, E. O'Neill, C. Westbury, and G. Frampton. 1999. "Home Visits by an Occupational Therapist for Assessment and Modification of Environmental Hazards: A Randomized Trial of Falls Prevention." *Journal of the American Geriatrics Society* 47, no. 12: 1397–1402.

Dunn, J. E., M. A. Rudberg, S. E. Furner, and C. K. Cassel. 1992. "Mortality, Disability, and Falls in Older Persons: The Role of Underlying Disease and Disability." *American Journal of Public Health* 82: 395–400.

Eisenberg, J. 2004. "Your Role in Fall Prevention." *Review of Optometry* (December 15): 46–50.

Ernst, F. R., and A. J. Grizzle. 2001. "Drug-Related Morbidity and Mortality: Updating the Cost-of-Illness Model." *Journal of the American Pharmaceutical Association* 41: 192–99.

Fleming, K. C., et al. 1993. "Shared Risk Factors for Falls, Incontinence, and Functional Dependence." *British Journal of General Practice* 43: 406–409.

FORE (Foundation for Osteoporosis Research and Education). 2007. "Osteoporosis and Osteopenia: Just the Facts." http://www.fore.org/patients/osteo_and_osteo-p2.html (accessed April 12, 2007).

Friedmann, P. D., L. Jin, T. Karrison, M. Nerney, D. Hayley, R. Mulliken, J. Walter, A. Miller, and M. Chin. 1999. "The Effect of Alcohol Abuse on the Health Status of Older Adults Seen in the Emergency Department." *American Journal of Drug and Alcohol Abuse* 25. http://www.questia.com/googleScholar.qst?docId=5001920818 (accessed May 13, 2008).

Fuller, G. F. 2000. "Falls in the Elderly." *American Family Physician* 61, no. 7: 2159–68, 2173–74.

Genant, H. K., C. Cooper, G. Poor, et al. 1999. "Interim Report and Recommendations of the World Health Organization Task-Force for Osteoporosis." *Osteoporosis International* 10: 259–64.

Gill, J., J. H. J. Allum, M. G. Carpenter, M. Held-Ziolkowska, A. L. Adkin, F. Honegger, and K. Pierchala. 2001. "Trunk Sway Measures of Postural Stability during Clinical Balance Tests Effects of Age." *Journals of*

Gerontology Series A: Biological Sciences and Medical Sciences 56: M438–M447.

Gleckman, R., and D. Hibert. 1982. "Afebrile Bacteremia. A Phenomenon in Geriatric Patients." *Journal of the American Medical Association* 248, no. 12: 1478–81.

Greenhouse, A. H. 1994. "Falls among the Elderly." In *Clinical Neurology of Aging*, 2nd ed. Edited by M. L. Albert and J. E. Knoefel, 611–26. New York: Oxford University Press.

Heoing, H. M., and L. Z. Rubenstein. 1991. "Hospital Associated Deconditioning and Dysfunction." *Journal of the American Geriatrics Society* 39: 220–22.

HHS. (US Department of Health and Human Services). 1996. *Physical Activity and Health: A Report of the Surgeon General.* Atlanta, GA: Centers for Disease Control and Prevention, National Center for Chronic Disease Prevention and Health Promotion.

———. 2004. "Bone Health and Osteoporosis: A Report of the Surgeon General."

Horikawa, E., T. Matsui, and H. Arai. 2005. "Risk of Falls in Alzheimer's Disease: A Prospective Study." *Internal Medicine* 44 no. 7 (July): 717–21.

Hwang, W., W. Weller, H. Ireys, and G. Anderson. 2001. "Out-of-Pocket Medical Spending for Care of Chronic Conditions." *Health Affairs* 20, no. 6 (November/December): 267–78. http://www.partnershipfor solutions.org/statistics/publications.html (accessed April 4, 2006).

Jackson, B. 2002. "Protecting the Elderly From Falls." *Chicago Tribune.* March 29. http://www.nsc.org/news/bj032902.htm (accessed January 21, 2007).

Jellinger, K. A. 2004. "Head Injury and Dementia." *Current Opinions in Neurology* 17, no. 6 (December): 719–23.

Kiel, D. P., P. O'Sullivan, and J. M. Teno. 1991. "Mortality vs. Health Care Utilization and Functional Status in the Aged Following a Fall." *Medical Care* 29. 221–28.

Kutner, N., H. Barnhart, and S. Wolf. 1997. "Self-Report Benefits of Tai Chi Practice by Older Adults." *Journal of Gerontology* 52, no. 5: 2422–46.

Leibson, C. L., A. N. A. Toteson, S. E. Gabriel, J. E. Ransom, and L. J. Melton. 2002. "Mortality, Disability, and Nursing Home Use for Persons with and without Hip Fracture: A Population-Based Study." *Journal of the American Geriatrics Society* 50: 1644–50.

Li, W., T. Keegan, B. Sternfeld, S. Sidney, C. Quesenberry Jr., and J. Kelsey. 2005. "Outdoor Falls among Middle-Aged and Older Adults: A Neglected Public Health Problem." *American Journal of Public Health* (October 21). http://www.ajph.org/cgi/content/abstract/AJPH.2005 .083055v1 (accessed February 6, 2007).

McGowan, J. 2003. *Word on Health.* December. http://www.nih.gov/news/ WordonHealth/dec2003/osteo.htm (accessed January 29, 2007).

McLaughlin, M. A., G. M. Orosz, J. Magaziner, E. L. Hannan, T. McGinn, R. S. Morrison, T. Hochman, K. Koval, M. Gilbert, and A. L. Siu. 2006. "Preoperative Status and Risk of Complications in Patients with Hip Fracture." *Journal of General Internal Medicine* 21 (March): 219–25.

Maki, B. E., and W. E. McIlroy. 2003. "Effects of Aging on Control of Stability." In *A Textbook of Audiological Medicine: Clinical Aspects of Hearing and Balance*, 671–90. London: Marin Dunitz Publishers.

Marcantonio, E. R., J. M. Flacker, R. J. Wright, and N. M. Resnick. 2001. "Reducing Delirium after Hip Fracture: A Randomized Trial." *Journal of the American Geriatrics Society* 49, no. 5 (May): 516–22.

Merck. 2005. *Merck Manual of Geriatrics.* Chapter 20, "Falls." http:// www.merck.com/mrkshared/mmg/sec2/ch20/ch20a.jsp (accessed January 29, 2007).

———. *Merck Manuals Online Medical Library.* "Osteoarthritis." http://www .merck.com/mmhe/sec05/ch066/ch066a.html (accessed January 13, 2007).

Mortimer, J. A., L. R. French, J. T. Hutton, and L. M. Schuman. 1985. "Head Injury as a Risk Factor for Alzheimer's Disease." *Neurology* 35, no. 2 (February): 264–67.

Mühlberg, W., and D. Platt. 1999. "Age-Dependent Changes of the Kidneys; Pharmacological Implications." *Gerontology* 45: 243–53.

NIAMS (National Institute of Arthritis and Musculoskeletal and Skin Diseases). 2005. "Preventing Falls and Related Fractures." http://www .niams.nih.gov/bone/hi/prevent_falls.htm (accessed February 2, 2007).

NIH (National Institutes of Health). 2000. "Osteoporosis Prevention, Diagnosis, and Therapy." *NIH Consensus Statement* 17: 1–45.

———. 2002. National Heart Lung and Blood Institute. "New Recommendations to Prevent High Blood Pressure Issued: Additional Lifestyle Approaches Advised." October 15.

NOF (National Osteoporosis Foundation). 1999. "Physician's Guide to Prevention and Treatment of Osteoporosis," pp. 1–9.

Ott, S. 2005. "Clinical Features of Osteoporosis." June 30. http://www
.courses.washington.edu/bonephys/opclin.html (accessed January 8,
2007).

RAND. 2003. "Evidence Report and Evidence-Based Recommendations:
Fall Prevention Interventions in the Medicare Population." Contract no.
500-98-0281.

Rubenstein, L. Z. 1993. "Falls." In *Ambulatory Geriatric Care*. Edited by T.
T. Yoshikawa, E. L. Cobbs, and K. Brummel-Smith, 296–304. St. Louis:
Mosby.

Samelson, E. J., Y. Zhang, and D. P. Kiel. 2002. "Effect of Birth Cohort on
Risk of Hip Fracture: Age-Specific Incidence Rates in the Framingham
Study." *American Journal of Public Health* 92, no. 5: 858–62.

SAMHSA (Substance Abuse & Mental Health Services Administration).
2007. "Prevention of Alcohol Misuse for Older Adults." Professional
Reference Series: *Alcohol Misuse Prevention, Volume 1*. http://www
.samhsa.gov/OlderAdultsTAC/docs/Alcohol_Booklet.pdf (accessed
April 13, 2007).

Schmucker, D. L. 2001. "Liver Function and Phase 1 Drug Metabolism in the
Elderly." *Drugs and Aging* 18: 837–51.

Scott, J. C. 1990. "Osteoporosis and Hip Fractures." *Rheumatic Diseases
Clinics of North America 1990* 16, no. 3: 717–40.

Scott, V., S. Peck, and P. Kendall. 2004. "Prevention of Falls and Injuries
among the Elderly: A Special Report from the Office of the Provincial
Health Officer."

SG (Surgeon General). 2004. *Bone Health and Osteoporosis: A Report of the
Surgeon General*. Chapter 5, "The Burden of Bone Disease." http://
www.surgeongeneral.gov/library/bonehealth/chapter_5.html#Direct
Costs (accessed April 13, 2007).

Simon, J., M. Leboff, J. Wright, and J. Glowacki. 2002. "Fractures in the
Elderly and Vitamin D." *Journal of Nutrition, Health and Aging* 6, no. 6:
406–12

Siu, A. L., J. D. Penrod, K. S. Boockvar, K. Koval, E. Strauss, and S. Morrison. 2006. "Early Ambulation after Hip Fracture: Effects on Function
and Mortality." *Archives of Internal Medicine* 166 (April): 766–71.

Sterling, D. A., J. A. O'Connor, and J. Bonadies. 2001. "Geriatric Falls:
Injury Severity Is High and Disproportionate to Mechanism." *Journal of
Trauma-Injury, Infection and Critical Care* 50, no. 1: 116–19.

Stevens, J. A., P. S. Corso, E. A. Finkelstein, and T. R. Miller. 2006. "The Costs of Fatal and Nonfatal Falls among Older Adults." *Injury Prevention* 12: 290–95.

Thorpe, K. 2004. "Hip Protectors to Reduce the Incidence of Hip Fractures in Older Persons." http://www.otcats.com/topics/CAT-Kathy_Thorp.pdf (accessed April 8, 2007).

Tinetti, M. E. 2003. "Clinical Practice. Preventing Falls in Elderly Persons." *New England Journal of Medicine* 348: 42–49.

Tinetti, M. E., W. L. Liu, and E. B. Claus. 1993. "Predictors and Prognosis of Inability to Get Up after Falls among Elderly Persons." *Journal of the American Medical Association* 269: 65–70.

Tinetti, M. E., M. Speechley, and S. F. Ginter. 1988. "Risk Factors for Falls among Elderly Persons Living in the Community." *New England Journal of Medicine* 319, no. 26: 1701–1707.

Vellas, B. J., S. J. Wayne, L. J. Romero, R. N. Baumgartner, and P. J. Garry. 1997. "Fear of Falling and Restriction of Mobility in Elderly Fallers." *Age and Ageing* 26: 189–93.

Verbrugge, L. M., and L. Juarez. 2001. "Profile of Arthritis Disability." *Public Health Report* 116, suppl. 1: 157–79.

Volkow, N. D., G. J. Wang, H. Begleiter, R. Hitzemann, N. Pappas, G. Burr, K. Pascani, C. Wong, J. Fowler, and A. Wolf. 1995. "Regional Brain Metabolic Response to Lorazepam in Subjects at Risk for Alcoholism." *Alcoholism: Clinical and Experimental Research* 19, no. 2: 510–16.

Weissman, D. E. 2000. "Pain Management for Patients with Late-Stage Dementia." HealthLink, Medical College of Wisconsin. http://www.healthlink.mcw.edu/article/967581724.html (accessed April 13, 2007).

Wolf, S. L., H. X. Barnhart, N. G. Kutner, E. McNeely, C. Coogler, and T. Xu. 1996. "Reducing Frailty and Falls in Older Persons: An Investigation of Tai Chi and Computerized Balance Training." *Journal of the American Geriatrics Society* 44, no. 5: 489–97.

Zeeh, J., and D. Platt. 2002. "The Aging Liver: Structural and Functional Changes and Their Consequences for Drug Treatment in Old Age." *Gerontology* 48, no. 3: 121–27.

CHAPTER 8

AA (Alzheimer's Association). 2008. Glossary entry. http://www.alz.org/carefinder/support/glossary.asp (accessed June 5, 2008).

AHCJ (Association of Health Care Journalists). 2002. *Covering the Quality of Health Care—A Resource Guide for Journalists.* Chapter 3, "Chronic Illness, Why It Matters: Huge Problem, Fascinating Questions." http://www.healthjournalism.org/qualityguide/chapter3.html#top (accessed March 5, 2007).

AHRQ (Agency for Healthcare Research and Quality). 2003. "Advanced Care Planning: Preferences for Care at the End of Life." *Research in Action* 12. March.

American Bar Association, Division of Public Education. 2007. "Law for Older Americans: Health Care Advance Directives." http://www.abanet.org/publiced/practical/patient_self_determination_act.html (accessed March 1, 2007).

Broadwell, A., E. V. Boisaubin, J. K. Dunn, and H. T. Engelhardt. 1993. "Advance Directives on Hospital Admission: A Survey of Patient Attitudes." *Southern Medical Journal* 86: 165–68.

CDC (Centers for Disease Control and Prevention) and HHS (Department of Health and Human Services). 2007. "Aging: End of Life Issues." January 16.

Donaldson, M., and M. J. Field. 1998. "Measuring Quality of Care at the End of Life." *Archives of Internal Medicine* 158: 121–28.

English, D. 2001. "The Uniform Health Care Decisions Act and Its Progress in the States." *Probate and Property.* May/June; updated February 2007. http://www.abanet.org/rppt/publications/magazine/2001/01mj/01mjenglish.html (accessed March 7, 2007)

FTC (Federal Trade Commission). 1994. "Facts for Business: Complying with the Funeral Rule." http://www.ftc.gov/bcp/conline/pubs/buspubs/funeral.htm#norequire (accessed March 14, 2007).

Hammes, B. J., and B. L. Rooney. 1998. "Death and End-of-Life Planning in One Midwestern Community." *Archives of Internal Medicine* 158: 383–90

Hanson, L. C., J. A. Tulsky, and M. Danis. 1997. "Can Clinical Interventions Change Care at the End of Life?" *Annals of Internal Medicine* 126: 381–88.

HHS (US Department of Health and Human Services). 2003. *Characteristics of Hospice Care Discharges and Their Length of Service: United States, 2000*. National Center for Health Statistics Series report 13, no. 154. http://www.cdc.gov/nchs/data/series/sr_13/sr13_154.pdf (accessed May 21, 2008).

Hyland, W. F., and D. S. Baime. 1976. "In Re Quinlan: A Synthesis of Law and Medical Technology." *Rutgers Camden Law Journal* 8, no. 1 (Fall): 37–64.

Kaufman, S. 2005. Excerpt from *And a Time to Die: How American Hospitals Shape the End of Life*. www.press.uchicago.edu/Misc/Chicago/426858.html (accessed February 26, 2007).

Kurent, J. 2000. "Death and Dying in America: The Need to Improve End-of-Life Care." *Carolina Healthcare Business*. http://www.ahcpr.gov/clinic/ptsafety/chap49.htm (accessed April 2, 2007).

Lynn, J. 2000. "Learning to Care for People with Chronic Illness Facing the End of Life." *Journal of the American Medical Association* 284, no. 19 (November 15): 2508–11.

McGlynn, E. A., S. M. Asch, and J. Adams. 2003. "The Quality of Health Care Delivered to Adults in the United States." *New England Journal of Medicine* 348, no. 26 (June 26): 2635–45.

Momeyer, R. 1990. "Finally, Let's Admit Nancy Cruzan Is Dead." *Newsday*, April 16.

Morrison, R. S., E. Olson, K. R. Mertz, and D. E. Meier. 1995. "The Inaccessibility of Advance Directives on Transfer from Ambulatory to Acute Care Settings." *Journal of the American Medical Association* 274: 478–82.

Nolo. 2008. Glossary entry. http://www.nolo.com/definition.cfm/term/2F667CEF-AEE9-4077-BCEA63652CADFDCD.

Poncy, M. 2006. "Ethics and Futile Care. Program and Abstracts of the National Conference of Gerontological Nurse Practitioners 25th Annual Meeting." September 27–October 1. http://www.medscape.com/viewarticle/550278 (accessed April 2, 2007).

Rao, J. K., J. Alongi, L. A. Anderson, L. Jenkins, G. A. Stokes, and M. Kane. 2005. "Development of Public Health Priorities for End-of-Life Initiatives." *American Journal of Preventive Medicine* 29, no. 5: 453–60.

Rao, J. K., L. A. Anderson, and S. M. Smith. 2002. "End of Life Is a Public Health Issue." *American Journal of Preventive Medicine* 23, no. 3: 215–20.

Sachs, G. A., J. Shega, D. Cox-Hayley. 2004. "Barriers to Excellent End-of-Life Care for Patients with Dementia." *Journal of General Internal Medicine* 19, no. 10 (October): 1057–63.

Schulz, R., and S. R. Beach. 1999. "Caregiving as a Risk Factor for Mortality: The Caregiver Health Effects Study." *Journal of the American Medical Association* 282, no. 23: 2259–60.

Shojania, K. G. 2001. "Making Health Care Safer: A Critical Analysis of Patient Safety Practices. Evidence Report/Technology Assessment." *Agency for Healthcare Research and Quality.* July. http://ahrq.hhs.gov/clinic/ptsafety/chap49.htm (accessed May 14, 2008).

Stern, D. 2006. "Advance Care Planning: The Time Is Now." *Vital Signs.* Member Publication of the Massachusetts Medical Society. http://www.massmed.org/AM/Template.cfm?Section=vs_nov06_Public_Health&TEMPLATE=/CM/ContentDisplay.cfm&CONTENTID=17444 (accessed March 15, 2007).

Teno, J., J. Lynn, N. Wenger, R. S. Phillips, D. P. Murphy, A. F. Connors Jr., N. Desbiens, W. Fulkerson, P. Bellamy, and W. A. Knaus. 1997. "Advance Directives for Seriously Ill Hospitalized Patients: Effectiveness with the Patient Self-Determination Act and the SUPPORT Intervention. SUPPORT Investigators. Study to Understand Prognoses and Preferences for Outcomes and Risks of Treatment." *Journal of the American Geriatrics Society* 45: 500–507.

Thompson, T., R. Barbour, and L. Schwartz. 2003. "Adherence to Advance Directives in Critical Care Decision Making: Vignette Study." *British Medical Journal* 327 (November): 1011.

Tsevat, J., E. F. Cook, M. L. Green, D. B. Matchar, N. V. Dawson, S. K. Broste, A. W. Wu, R. S. Phillips, R. K. Oye, and L. Goldman. 1995. "Health Values of the Seriously Ill." *Annals of Internal Medicine* 122: 514–20.

Tsevat, J., N. V. Dawson, A. W. Wu, J. Lynn, J. R. Soukup, E. F. Cook, H. Vidaillet, and R. S. Phillips. 1998. "Health Values of Hospitalized Patients 80 Years or Older." *Journal of the American Medical Association* 279: 371–75.

Ulferts, A., A. Kumar, and W. Levesque. 2005. "U. S. House Acts to Save Schiavo." *St. Petersburg Times.* March 17. http://www.sptimes.com/2005/03/17/Tampabay/US_House_acts_to_save.shtml (accessed February 26, 2007).

Wissow, L., A. Belote, W. Kramer, A. Compton-Phillips, R. Kritzler, and J. Weiner. 2004. "Promoting Advance Directives among Elderly Primary Care Patients." *Journal of General Internal Medicine* 19, no. 9 (September): 944–51.

INDEX

Increasingly, research consistently shows that lower-fat diets in young and middle-aged adults may reduce the risk for AD decades later. Not all fat is bad, however. Some fats may benefit brain health. One study found that a Mediterranean diet high in olive oil is protective against age-related cognitive decline (Solfrizzi et al. 1999). This might also be true for other unsaturated vegetable oils.

Activities

Physical activity has the ability to improve blood flow to the brain, reduce cardiovascular risk factors, and may also stimulate nerve cell growth and survival. One study of healthy adults between ages sixty and seventy-five revealed mental activities involving planning, scheduling, monitoring, and memory improved in a group participating in aerobic exercise (Small 2002).

Regular exercise to keep hearts healthy has long been recommended by physicians. Along with cardiovascular benefits, new evidence is showing that people who are active during their middle years seem to be at a much lower risk for dementia, particularly AD. Scientists have learned that middle-aged people who exercised at least twice a week had a 50 percent lower chance of developing dementia and a 60 percent lower chance of developing AD than their sedentary peers. The exercise reported was mostly walking and biking strenuously enough to cause sweating and strained breathing.

Another unexpected conclusion of the research was that exercise was found to be most beneficial for those individuals who were predisposed to dementia and AD (Kivipelto et al. 2006). Again, there is evidence that if certain lifestyle habits are identified and treated in middle age, then the prospect of avoiding dementia increases.

Using Medications

As mentioned earlier, high levels of blood cholesterol are a known risk factor for heart disease and there are indications these high levels are also